Color Atlas of
Gonioscopy

Wallace L. M. Alward, *MD*

Associate Professor of Ophthalmology
Director of Glaucoma Service
Department of Ophthalmology
The University of Iowa
Iowa City

Illustrated by:

Lee Allen
Associate Emeritus
Department of Ophthalmology
The University of Iowa
Iowa City

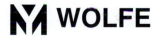 WOLFE

To my wife
Kazi
and children
Alec, Sarah, and Erin
for their love and patience

Copyright © 1994 Mosby–Year Book Europe Limited. Copyright for Figures **137, 184, 241, 261, 262** and **265** is held by Abbott Laboratories, North Chicago, Illinois.
Published in1994 by Wolfe Publishing, an imprint of Mosby–Year Book Europe Limited
Printed by Grafos, S.A. ARTE SOBRE PAPEL, Barcelona
ISBN 0 7234 1790 3

For full details of all Mosby–Year Book Europe Limited titles please write to Mosby–Year Book Europe Limited, Lynton House, 7–12 Tavistock Square, London WC1H 9LB, England.

A CIP catalogue record for this book is available from the British Library.

Library of Congress Cataloging-in-Publication Data *(applied for)*

Contents

Foreword

It is indeed a pleasure to write an introduction to this new and splendid gonioscopic atlas. It has been decades since such an atlas has appeared in this country. The old versions are now obsolete and out of print. A new one is badly needed and this represents a welcome addition to our basic material for learning and teaching.

Dr Alward, the chief of our Glaucoma Service, has a rich clinical experience, which, combined with a profound basic knowledge and an investigative curiosity, has provided him with all the necessary attributes to write such a text and to collect these hundreds of beautiful photographs. They are of excellent didactic value and will be studied with advantage by neophyte and expert alike.

In addition to the photographs, Dr Alward was able to incorporate the original paintings made by Mr Lee Allen. These pictures were created many years ago and were originally requested by Dr Walter Benedict on behalf of the American Academy of Ophthalmology and Otolaryngology. The project was never realized and the drawings lingered in a storage room until Dr Alward resurrected them. The illustrations juxtapose in a perfect manner the clinical appearance and the histologic substrate. Lee Allen, this man of many talents, has proven here once again that he is a master of the visual arts as applied to opthalmology.

We are all indebted to Dr Alward for collating this rich material, for writing the informative text, for taking and collecting the many photographs of the chamber angle, and for rescuing the beautiful drawings of Lee Allen from oblivion. May the book find the general acceptance it so richly deserves.

Frederick C. Blodi, MD
Department of Ophthalmology
The University of Iowa Hospital and Clinics
Iowa City, Iowa

Preface

Gonioscopy is an integral part of any complete ophthalmic examination. Unfortunately, techniques for viewing the angle can initially seem difficult. When the angle is seen, its appearance may be confusing. The goal of this atlas is to provide a brief, but comprehensive, introduction to gonioscopy. Gonioscopy is a visual science, so the greater part of the book is devoted to illustrations of gonioscopic and slit-lamp findings, normal and abnormal.

I was inspired to write this book when I discovered a remarkable collection of watercolor paintings of the angle created by Lee Allen in the late 1940s and early 1950s. I feel that these paintings show the angle with a unique clarity. Photographs of the angle often sacrifice detail for panorama or panorama for detail; paintings are able to include both. The corneal wedge is a very helpful landmark in studying the angle, which does not photograph well. Mr. Allen has used the corneal wedge to aid our interpretation of these paintings. I have used his paintings to illustrate points whenever possible and have used photographs when no paintings were available.

Lee Allen is uniquely qualified to bring us such images of the angle. He has been an accomplished artist since his teens, spending his early career working closely with the noted American artist Grant Wood. He was medical illustrator for the Department of Ophthalmology at the University of Iowa for over 40 years. During this time he developed a direct goniolens (Allen, 1944), the Allen gonioprism (Allen and O'Brien, 1945), and the Allen–Thorpe four-mirror gonioprism (Allen et al., 1954). He studied the anatomy and embryology of the angle and published extensively on the subject (Allen and Burian, 1965; Allen et al., 1955; Braley and Allen, 1954; Burian and Allen, 1961; Burian et al., 1954, 1957). With Dr Hermann Burian he developed trabeculotomy ab externo for infantile glaucoma (Allen and Burian, 1961, 1962). Lee Allen has a number of other accomplishments in ophthalmology that are not related to glaucoma. His contributions to photography include the Allen Separator for stereo photography of the fundus and the Allen Dot to remove aberrations from fundus photographs (Allen, 1964a, 1964b; Braley and Allen, 1951; Douvas and Allen, 1950; Von Noorden et al., 1959). He was a pioneer in fluorescein angiography, particularly of the anterior segment. Lee was a founding member of the American Society of Ocularists and has contributed the Allen, Iowa, and Universal implants to that field (Allen and Allen, 1950; Allen et al., 1960; O'Brien et al., 1946). He developed the Burian–Allen electroretinogram electrode (Burian and Allen, 1954). He has also published on mechanisms of accommodation (Burian and Allen, 1955) and on instrumentation for penetrating keratoplasty (Lee and Allen, 1949; Watzke and Allen, 1963). Lee Allen serves as a model of ingenuity and dedication. His accomplishments are especially impressive because he had no formal medical training. The *Journal of Ophthalmic Photography* devoted one recent issue to his remarkable career (Wong and Fishman, 1990).

This is an atlas of gonioscopy, not a comprehensive textbook of glaucoma. Many excellent glaucoma textbooks are available. I have resisted the urge to discuss treatment of the pathological processes mentioned, referring readers instead to the excellent textbooks of Shields (1992), Hoskins and Kass (1989), Epstein (1986), and Ritch, Shields and Krupin (1989) for further information about the diseases described.

Acknowledgments

I am grateful for the help and support that I have received from the faculty and staff of the Department of Ophthalmology at the University of Iowa. Paul M. Munden, MD, John A. Campagna, MD, and William L. Haynes, MD, of the Glaucoma Service helped review segments of the book and provided helpful advice. My secretary, Peg Harris, was a great help in this endeavor. Our departmental photographic service was invaluable: Ray Northway, Joanne Montgomery, and Ed Heffron deserve particular mention.

I thank Douglas R. Anderson, MD, Paul Palmberg, MD, Ph.D, Elizabeth A. Hodapp, MD, and Richard K. Parrish II, MD, of The Bascom Palmer Eye Institute, Miami, Florida, for teaching me about glaucoma and gonioscopy.

I would like to thank all of those who allowed me to use their illustrations for this work. They are acknowledged in the captions to individual illustrations. Robert Ritch, MD, Paul R. Lichter, MD, and A. Tim Johnson, M.D, Ph.D, have been especially generous.

James Erickson and Phillip Erickson of Ocular Instruments provided lenses for several of the illustrations.

Geoff Greenwood of Mosby–Year Book Europe has made writing this book a pleasure. He has always been supportive and encouraging.

A special thanks to Lee Allen for making available his original paintings and for coming out of retirement to do one more painting (Figure 274) after a hiatus of 40 years.

Some of the illustrations for the text, including Mr Allen's watercolors, photographs of gross pathology, and photomicrographs, appeared previously in the University of Iowa Videodisc Project II (Pathology of the Eye and Basic Ophthalmology). These illustrations are copyright 1991 and are used with the permission of the Department of Ophthalmology, University of Iowa, Iowa City, Iowa.

Figures **137, 184, 241, 251, 261, 262,** and **265** appeared in *What's New*, published by Abbott Laboratories, North Chicago, Illinois, in 1952, and are used with their permission.

Figures **184, 185** and **265** are correctly oriented, although the artist's name appears upside down.

1 Anatomy of the Angle

The purpose of gonioscopy is to permit visualization of the iridocorneal angle (or simply 'angle'). This is the area in which the trabecular meshwork lies and is therefore the part of the eye that is responsible for aqueous outflow. Before describing gonioscopic techniques and findings it is important to review briefly the anatomy and function of the structures of the angle (**1** and **2**).

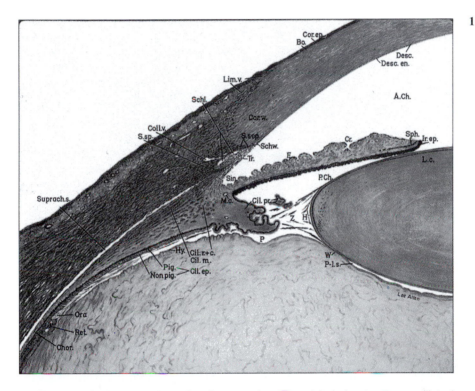

1

1 Sketch of the anterior chamber angle. The labeled structures (listed alphabetically) are: **A. Ch.**, anterior chamber; **Bo.**, Bowman's layer; **Chor.**, choroid; **Cil. ep.**, ciliary epithelium; **Cil. m.**, ciliary muscle (longitudinal); **Cil. pr.**, ciliary process; **Cil. r. + c.**, ciliary body (radial and circular muscles); **Coll. v.**, collector veins; **Cor. ep.**, corneal epithelium; **Cor. w.**, corneal wedge; **Cr.**, iris crypt; **Desc.**, Descemet's membrane; **Desc. en.**, corneal endothelium (or Descemet's endothelium); **F**, iris furrow; **H**, Hanover's canal; **Hy.**, hyaloid; **Ir. ep.**, iris pigment epithelium; **L. c.**, lens cortex; **Lim. v.**, limbal vessels; **M. c.**, major circle of iris; **Non pig.**, non-pigmented ciliary epithelium; **Ora**, ora serrata; **P**, Petit's canal; **Pig.**, pigmented ciliary epithelium; **P. Ch.**, posterior chamber; **P-l. s.**, post-lenticular space; **Ret.**, retina; **Schl.**, Schlemm's canal; **Schw.**, Schwalbe's line; **Sin.**, angle recess (or sinus); **Sph.**, sphincter; **S. sep.**, scleral septum; **S. sp.**, scleral spur; **Suprach. s.**, suprachoroidal space; **Tr.**, trabecular meshwork; **W**, Wieger's ligament; **Z**, zonules. (Because this sketch was drawn in the 1940s some of the terms, such as Descemet's endothelium, are different from those used today.)

2

3

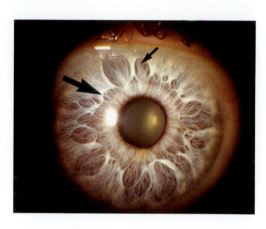

2 Histopathologic slide of the chamber angle showing structures labeled in **1**. Hematoxylin and eosin stain. (Courtesy of Robert Folberg, MD, University of Iowa.)

3 Normal iris. The peripheral ciliary zone is separated from the pupillary zone by the wavy collarette (large arrow). The narrow band of sphincter muscle can be seen around the pupil. This iris has many crypts (small arrow).

Iris

When examined with the slit lamp, the iris is seen to have two main zones – a central pupillary zone and a peripheral ciliary zone (**3**). These areas are separated by a wavy border, the collarette. There are intermittent crypts, which can extend deep into the stoma, and also concentric furrows, which become more prominent as the pupil dilates.

The iris is composed of an anterior stromal layer and a posterior epithelial layer. The stroma is vascular connective tissue that has no anterior epithelial covering. The musculature of the iris lies within the stroma. A 1 mm wide band of sphincter muscle rings the pupil. The myoepithelial cells of the dilator muscle are spread throughout the stroma from the iris root as far centrally as the sphincter. Blood vessels in the iris are mostly located in the stromal layer and have a radial orientation. They are frequently visible in lightly pigmented eyes. The greater circle of the iris is found in the ciliary body or in the root of the iris, and is occasionally visible in a gonioscopic examination.

Posteriorly, there are two epithelial layers. As in the ciliary body, the cells of these two epithelial layers are aligned apex to apex. The anterior layer has little pigmentation and is continuous with the outer (pigmented) layer of the ciliary body. The posterior layer is densely pigmented and faces the posterior chamber. This layer is continuous with the non-pigmented layer of ciliary epithelium.

The iris generally inserts at a variable level into the face of the ciliary body, posterior to the scleral spur. Less commonly, the iris will insert on, or anterior to, the scleral spur. The iris thins at the periphery near its insertion.

Ciliary Body Face

The ciliary body lies behind the iris. Its many functions include the manufacture of aqueous humor, the control of accommodation, the regulation of aqueous outflow, the secretion of hyaluronate into the vitreous, and maintenance of a portion of the blood–aqueous barrier. There are two major muscle groups in the ciliary body: the circular muscle fibers, which are responsible for accommodation, and the longitudinal muscle fibers, which control the outflow of aqueous by pulling open the trabecular meshwork and Schlemm's canal.

The ciliary body face is that portion of the ciliary body which borders on the anterior chamber. The degree to which the ciliary body face is visible depends on the level and angle of iris insertion. In some eyes the ciliary body face is not visible, being completely obscured by iris.

Although most outflow of aqueous occurs through the trabecular meshwork, approximately 10% is by non-conventional routes, primarily through the ciliary body face into the suprachoroidal space (Bill and Phillips, 1971). This uveoscleral outflow is pressure-independent.

Cholinergic agents, such as pilocarpine, compact the fibers in the ciliary body and decrease uveoscleral outflow. Anti-cholinergic drugs, such as atropine, increase non-conventional outflow through the ciliary body face (Bill and Phillips, 1971). In some eyes with severe compromise of trabecular outflow anti-cholinergic medications may lower intraocular pressure, while cholinergic drugs may, paradoxically, increase intraocular pressure. The prostaglandin $F_{2\alpha}$ drugs appear to promote a marked increase in non-conventional outflow through the ciliary body face (Gabelt and Kaufman, 1989). These drugs are currently being evaluated for a possible role in glaucoma therapy.

Scleral Spur

The scleral spur is composed of a ring of collagen fibers that run parallel to the limbus. It marks the posterior border of the trabecular meshwork. The spur projects slightly into the anterior chamber and is seen as a white to yellowish line in most eyes. The longitudinal muscle of the ciliary body attaches to the scleral spur and opens the trabecular meshwork by pulling on the spur. On histopathologic slides the scleral spur can be located by following the longitudinal muscle of the ciliary body forward to its point of attachment (4). The structural integrity supplied by the scleral spur may prevent the ciliary muscle from causing Schlemm's canal to collapse (Moses and Grodzki, 1977).

4   The scleral sulcus, in which the trabecular meshwork lies, is clearly demonstrated in this histopathological specimen stained with the Masson trichrome stain. The scleral sulcus is bordered anteriorly by Schwalbe's line (white arrow) and posteriorly by the scleral spur (black arrow). The longitudinal muscle (**LM**) of the ciliary body attaches to the scleral spur. The separation between sclera and ciliary body (∗) is an artifact. (Armed Forces Institute of Pathology.)

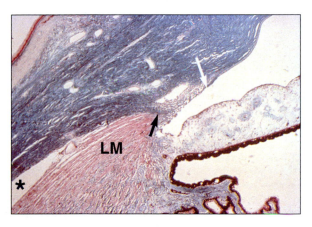

4

Trabecular Meshwork

The trabecular meshwork is located between the scleral spur and Schwalbe's line. Most of the trabecular meshwork sits within the scleral sulcus (**4**). Approximately 90% of aqueous outflow is through the trabecular meshwork. This flow is pressure-dependent, increasing as intraocular pressure increases. Aqueous humor flowing through the trabecular meshwork enters Schlemm's canal and from there flows into the scleral, episcleral, and conjunctival venous systems. For aqueous to exit the eye by this route, the intraocular pressure must be higher than the episcleral venous pressure. At pressures below episcleral venous pressure (8–15 mm Hg) all aqueous outflow must be via non-conventional routes (**5**) (Pederson, 1986).

The trabecular meshwork consists of three layers (**6**). Closest to the aqueous is the uveal meshwork, which consists of endothelium-coated collagen beams separated by large (25–75 μm)

spaces (**7**). The uveal meshwork extends from the ciliary body in the angle recess to Schwalbe's line and covers the ciliary body face, the scleral spur and the trabecular meshwork. In most eyes the uveal meshwork is colorless and is either not visible or is seen only as a glistening veil in the angle of young patients. In some eyes the uveal meshwork is dense and pigmented, giving a rough appearance to the trabecular meshwork and occasionally obscuring portions of the scleral spur. The uveal meshwork does not provide any resistance to aqueous outflow. Iris processes appear as thicker strands in front of the uveal meshwork and extend from the periphery of the iris to the trabecular meshwork (Chapter 5).

The next, deeper, layer – the corneoscleral meshwork – extends from the scleral spur to the anterior wall of the scleral sulcus. It is a layer of five to nine sheets of endothelium-coated collagen fibers perforated by holes of 5–50 μm

5

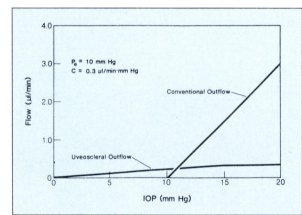

5 Uveoscleral and trabecular (conventional) outflow as a function of the intraocular pressure. Below episcleral venous pressure all outflow is through uveoscleral and other non-conventional means. **C**, outflow facility; **IOP**, intraocular pressure; P_e, episcleral venous pressure. (Jonathan E. Pederson, MD. Published courtesy of *Transactions of the Ophthalmological Society of the United Kingdom* 1986; **105:** 220–226.)

6

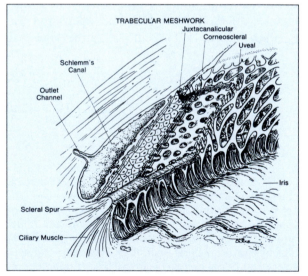

6 The three layers of the trabecular meshwork (uveal, corneoscleral, and juxtacanalicular) are shown in this cut-away illustration. (Published courtesy of M. Bruce Shields, MD, *Textbook of Glaucoma.* Williams and Wilkins, Baltimore, 1992.)

(Flocks, 1956). This layer, like the uveal meshwork, does not offer significant resistance to aqueous outflow.

The deepest layer of the trabecular meshwork is the juxtacanalicular tissue, the last layer that aqueous crosses before entering Schlemm's canal. The juxtacanalicular tissue has trabecular endothelium on one side and Schlemm's endothelium on the other. Between these endothelial layers is a loose connective tissue. This juxtacanalicular tissue provides the most resistance to aqueous outflow. The aqueous must travel through the endothelium of Schlemm's canal to enter the canal. There are no direct routes of any significance between endothelial cells into Schlemm's canal. Sondermann's canals have been described in the past as being direct passages through the juxtacanalicular tissue to Schlemm's canal, but there is doubt that such passages actually exist.

Aqueous outflow occurs primarily through the posterior portion of the trabecular meshwork – which is the portion that overlies Schlemm's canal. With time, this posterior portion of the meshwork usually becomes pigmented, whereas the anterior meshwork usually remains relatively non-pigmented.

The endothelial cells in the trabecular meshwork differ from corneal endothelial cells in that they are larger with less prominent cell borders (**8**) (Spencer *et al.*, 1968). A function of endothelial cells is to digest phagocytized foreign material. After engulfing foreign material some endothelial cells undergo autolysis or migrate away from the trabecular meshwork into Schlemm's canal (Grierson and Chisholm, 1978). With age or repeated insult the endothelial cell count decreases, as does aqueous outflow.

7

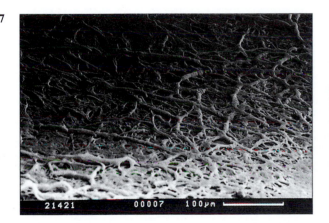

8

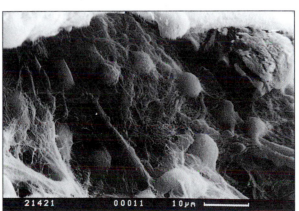

7 Pillars of the uveal trabecular meshwork are seen in this scanning electron micrograph. Note the large intervening spaces which do not provide resistance to aqueous outflow. (Courtesy of Carmen Rummelt and Volker Rummelt, MD, University of Erlangen–Nürnberg.)

8 Scanning electron micrograph of trabecular endothelial cells with large nuclei and indistinct cell borders. (Courtesy of Carmen Rummelt and Volker Rummelt, MD, University of Erlangen–Nürnberg.)

Schlemm's Canal

A 190–350 μm diameter tube at the base of the scleral sulcus, Schlemm's canal collects aqueous and drains it into the venous system (Hoffmann and Dumitrescu, 1971). Occasionally, the canal is a plexus rather than a single, discrete vessel. On the trabecular side of Schlemm's canal there are many vacuoles through which aqueous traverses the endothelial cells. The vacuoles and the prominent nuclei of the endothelial cells lining the trabecular side of the canal give it a roughened appearance (**9**) (Tripathi, 1968). On the scleral side of Schlemm's canal the endothelium is much smoother and is intermittently perforated by 25 to 35 aqueous collector channels.

Schlemm's canal is not a rigid structure, although it does contain septa, which provide some support. At high intraocular pressures the canal collapses and resistance to aqueous outflow increases. The longitudinal muscle of the ciliary body can open Schlemm's canal by pulling on the scleral spur. Cholinergic drugs may decrease resistance to outflow through this action.

Schwalbe's Line

Schwalbe's line occurs in a 50–150 μm transition zone (zone S) between the trabecular meshwork and the corneal endothelium (**10**). It is the anterior border of the trabecular meshwork and the posterior border of Descemet's membrane. There is also a transition from the scleral curvature to the steeper corneal curvature at Schwalbe's line, which can cause a settling of pigment in this area.

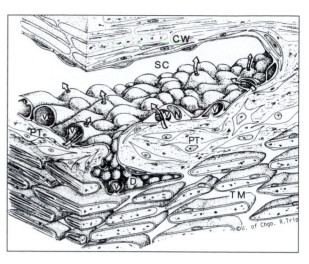

9 Schlemm's canal, demonstrating the roughened endothelial surface on the trabecular meshwork side of the canal and the smoother surface on the corneoscleral side of the canal. Aqueous passes through the endothelium and into Schlemm's canal by way of the vesicles. **CW**, corneoscleral wall; **D**, diverticulum; **PT**, pericanalicular connective tissue; **N**, nucleus of cell; **SC**, Schlemm's canal; **V**, vesicle. (Courtesy of Ramesh C. Tripathi, MD. In Frederick A. Jakobiec ed. *Ocular Anatomy, Embryology and Teratology.* Harper and Row, Philadelphia, 1982.)

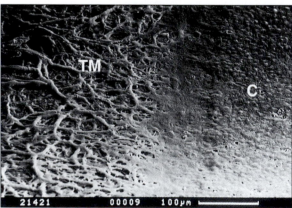

10 Schwalbe's line, demonstrating transition from trabecular meshwork endothelium (**TM**) to corneal endothelium (**C**). (Courtesy of Carmen Rummelt and Volker Rummelt, MD, University of Erlangen–Nürnberg.)

2 A Brief History of Gonioscopy

Gonioscopy is a relatively young science, having been developed entirely within the twentieth century.

The Greek ophthalmologist Alexios Trantas (**11**) first reported examination of the angle in 1907. He viewed the angle in a patient with keratoglobus using a direct ophthalmoscope while indenting the sclera with his finger (Trantas, 1907). Some years later he presented remarkably detailed drawings of the angle (**12**) (Trantas, 1918). He coined the term 'gonioscopy', meaning 'observation of the angle', from the Greek (Dellaporta, 1975).

Maximilian Salzmann (**13**) recognized that the normal angle was not visible owing to total internal reflection (Salzmann, 1914). He was the first to view the angle through a contact lens and, in 1915, presented a paper with excellent drawings of the angle obtained by means of his newly developed contact lens (Salzmann, 1915). Salzmann stressed the importance of gonioscopic examination in patients with a history of angle closure. He recognized that the development of synechiae in the angle did not always lead to elevated intraocular pressure. Salzmann was also the first to describe blood in Schlemm's canal.

Mizuo (1914) examined the inferior angle in patients by everting the lower lid and filling the cul-de-sac with saline. The technique was difficult to perform because the saline lens was lost when the patient blinked.

The introduction of Zeiss' slit lamp permitted significant advances in gonioscopy. Koeppe (1919) used the Zeiss slit lamp to examine the

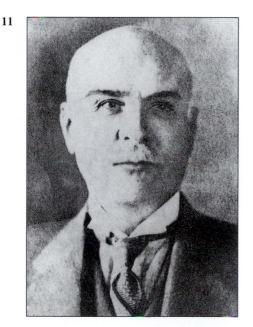

11 Alexios Trantas (1867–1961). (A. Dellaporta, MD. Published courtesy of *Survey of Ophthalmology* 1975; **20:** 137–149.)

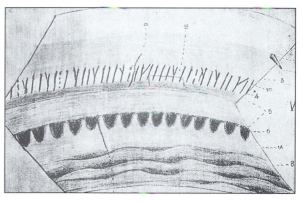

12 This drawing of the angle, made by Trantas in 1918, demonstrates remarkable detail. The angle was viewed with an ophthalmoscope while the limbus was indented by the examiner's finger. (A. Trantas, MD, L'Ophtalmoscopie de l'angle irido-cornéen (gonioscopie). *Archives d'ophtalmologie* (Paris) 1918; **36:** 257–276.)

angle with his newly developed lens, which was thicker and more convex than Salzmann's lens. Gonioscopy was performed with the patient seated at the slit lamp. A knotted bandage rested on a central depression in the lens to secure it to the patient. This technique was effective only for evaluating the nasal and temporal sectors of the angle.

In 1925 Manuel Uribe Troncoso developed a self-illuminating monocular gonioscope that permitted examination of all parts of the angle (Troncoso, 1925).

Thorburn was the first to photograph the angle. In 1927 he photographed an instance of angle closure brought on by mydriatics and subsequently reversed by eserine. He also observed that the majority of his patients with glaucoma had open angles (Thorburn, 1927).

Otto Barkan used a slit lamp suspended from the ceiling and a hand-held illuminator to view the angle through a Koeppe lens (Barkan *et al.*, 1936). His technique had the advantage of bright illumination and sufficient magnification, and his apparatus brought gonioscopy into practical clinical application. He subsequently made the distinction between 'deep-chamber' and 'shallow-chamber' glaucoma, and suggested that iridectomy be used for shallow-chamber glaucoma only (Barkan, 1938).

Barkan was also the first to describe goniotomy under direct visualization (Barkan, 1937).

Indirect gonioscopy was introduced with the Goldmann mirrored contact lens (Goldmann, 1938). The Allen lens, developed a few years later, used a totally refractive prism rather than a mirror (Allen and O'Brien, 1945). This was later modified into the Allen–Thorpe gonioprism, which had four prisms and permitted most of the angle to be viewed without rotation of the lens (Allen *et al.*, 1954).

The first attempt to grade the angle was that of Gradle and Sugar (1940). Scheie (1957) developed a grading system based on visible structures. The widely used Shaffer grading technique was developed three years later (Shaffer, 1960). This system was modified by Spaeth to provide information regarding the angle of iris approach, the level of iris insertion, and the configuration of the iris (Spaeth, 1971). The techniques of angle grading are described more completely in Chapter 6.

An excellent review of the history of gonioscopy has been provided by Dellaporta (1975).

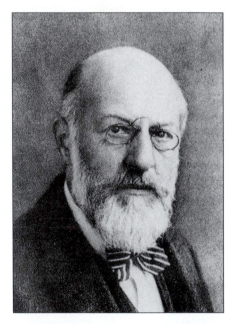

13 Maximilian Salzmann (1862–1954). (A. Dellaporta, MD. Published courtesy of *Survey of Ophthalmology* 1975; **20:** 137–149.)

3 Principles of Gonioscopy

It is not possible to view the anterior chamber of a normal eye directly (**14**). Light from the junction of the iris and cornea strikes the tear–air interface at a shallow angle and is totally reflected back into the eye (**15**). This principle of total internal reflection is used in the design of fiberoptic cables. If light from the interior of the eye strikes the cornea at an angle steeper than 46° (the critical angle), the light will exit the eye and the trabecular meshwork will be visible (Shields, 1992). Rarely, this may occur in eyes with keratoconus, keratoglobus, or severe myopia (**16**). The angle of approach to the trabecular meshwork can be altered if the limbus is indented, as shown by Trantas in his initial description of gonioscopy (**17**) (Trantas, 1907).

14

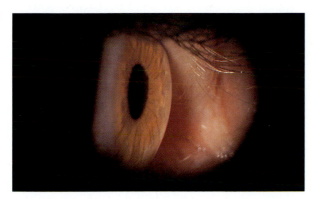

14 Slit-lamp view attempting to visualize the angle in a normal eye. No angle structures are visible because of total internal reflection.

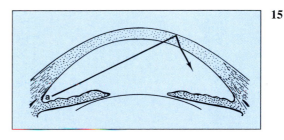

15

15 Light from the anterior chamber angle (**a**) undergoes total internal reflection at the tear–air interface and is not visible to the examiner.

16

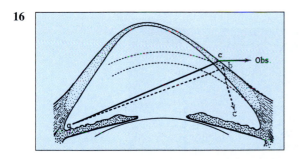

16 In an eye with keratoconus light from the trabecular meshwork (**a**) strikes the cornea at a steep enough angle to permit direct visualization of the trabecular meshwork by the observer (**Obs.**). This is an uncommon situation.

17

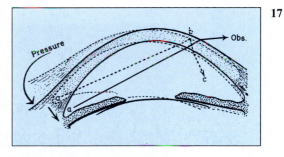

17 Indentation of the limbus brings angle structures (**a**) into direct view without a lens. It is very difficult to obtain an undistorted view in this manner.

In modern gonioscopy contact lenses are used to overcome the problem of total internal reflection.

Two basic types of lens are used: the direct lens and the indirect lens.

Direct Gonioscopy

Direct gonioscopy is performed with a steeply convex lens, which permits light from the angle to exit the eye closer to the perpendicular at the interface between the lens and the air (**18**). The Koeppe lens (**19** and **20**), which is a 50-diopter lens, is placed on the eye of a recumbent patient using saline to bridge the gap between lens and cornea (**21**). The examiner views the angle through a hand-held binocular microscope, which is counterbalanced to permit ease of handling. Illumination is provided by a light source that is held in the other hand (**22**). The Koeppe lens magnifies ×1.5. This, in combination with the ×16 magnification of the oculars, yields a total magnification of ×24. Koeppe lenses are manufactured in several sizes to suit infants to adults.

18

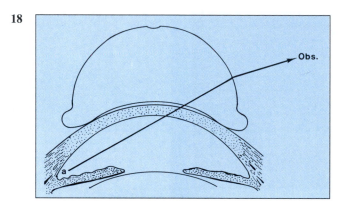

18 Direct gonioscopic lenses change the angle of the interface with the air so that the light from the trabecular meshwork (**a**) exits more perpendicularly.

19 **20**

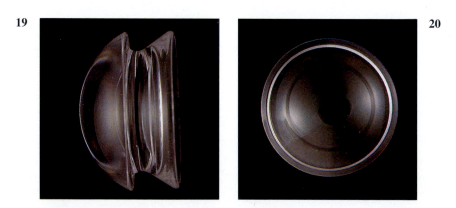

19, 20 The Koeppe lens for direct gonioscopy is available in several sizes. (Courtesy of Ocular Instruments.)

Direct lenses are used for surgical procedures such as goniotomy and goniosynechialysis. The Hoskins–Barkan (**23** and **24**) and Swan–Jacobs (**25** and **26**) lenses are most commonly used in the operating room. These lenses can also be used to examine sedated infants with an operating microscope or with a portable slit lamp (**27** and **28**).

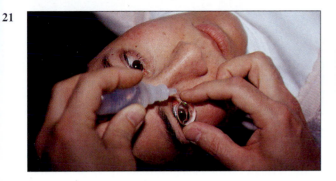

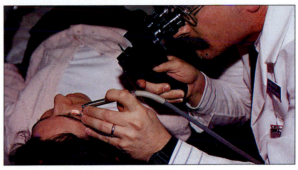

21 Saline is used to bridge the gap between the Koeppe lens and the cornea in a supine patient. (Courtesy of Paul R. Lichter, MD, and A. Tim Johnson, MD, Ph.D, University of Michigan.)

22 Examination of supine patient with Koeppe lens using counterbalanced biomicroscope and Barkan illuminator. (Courtesy of Paul R. Lichter, MD, and A. Tim Johnson, MD, Ph.D, University of Michigan.)

23, 24 Hoskins–Barkan surgical contact lens. This direct lens is used with loupes or an operating microscope for goniotomy and other angle surgery. (Courtesy of Ocular Instruments.)

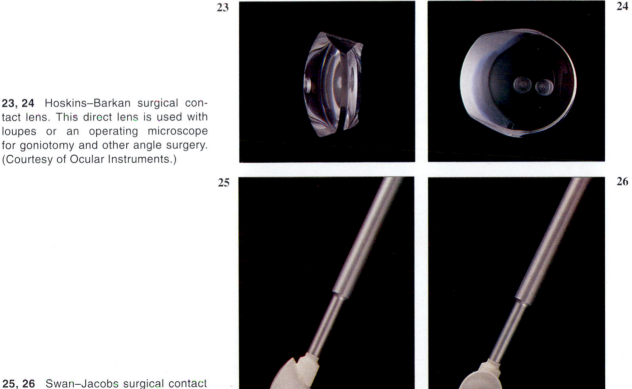

25, 26 Swan–Jacobs surgical contact lens. This direct lens is used with loupes or an operating microscope for goniotomy and other angle surgery. (Courtesy of Ocular Instruments.)

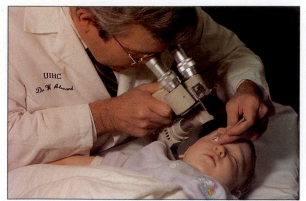

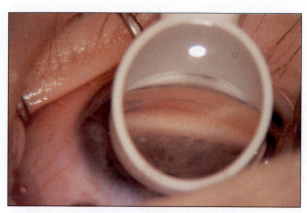

27 Gonioscopy can be performed on sedated infants with a direct contact lens and an operating microscope or a portable slit lamp. Here a Swan–Jacobs lens is used with a portable slit lamp to examine the eye of a sedated child with primary infantile glaucoma.

28 View through a Swan–Jacobs lens into the angle of a child with primary infantile glaucoma.

Indirect Gonioscopy

The lenses used in indirect gonioscopy use mirrors to overcome total internal reflection. The mirror redirects light from the angle so that it exits the eye perpendicularly to the lens–air interface (**29**). The examination is performed at the slit lamp and takes advantage of the latter's flexible illumination and magnification system.

The Goldmann three-mirror lens (**30** and **31**) has a mirror through which the angle is viewed. There are two additional mirrors for examination of the peripheral retina. The Goldmann lens is coupled to the cornea by means of a viscous methylcellulose fluid. The lens has a broad (12 mm) area of contact with the globe and can, under the application of pressure, artificially close the angle or reflux blood into Schlemm's canal. The single-mirror Goldmann lens has only the gonioscopic mirror (**32** and **33**). The Ritch trabeculoplasty laser lens (**34** and **35**) is similar to the Goldmann lens except that all four of its

29
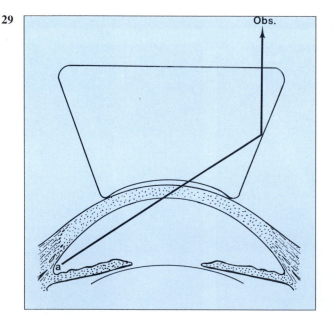
Obs.

29 Indirect gonioscopic lenses use mirrors or prisms to reflect the light from the irido-corneal angle (**a**) so that it leaves the eye perpendicular to the face of the contact lens.

30 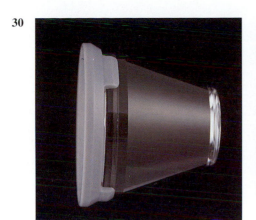 31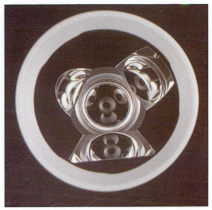

30, 31 Goldmann three-mirror lens. The shortest mirror is for examining the angle. The other two mirrors are for examining the peripheral retina. Like all indirect lenses, the central area can be used to examine the fundus. (Haag-Streit.)

32 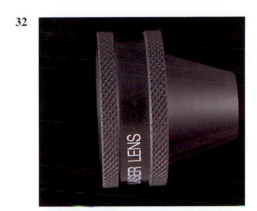 33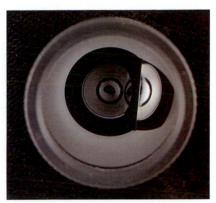

32, 33 Goldmann style one-mirror lens. (Courtesy of Ocular Instruments.)

34 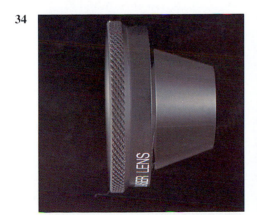 35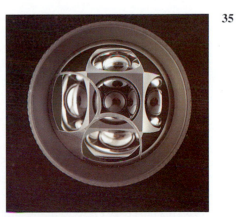

34, 35 Ritch trabeculoplasty laser lens. Two 59° mirrors are designed to view the inferior angle and two 64° mirrors are designed to view the superior angle. A convex button in front of one 59° mirror and one 64° mirror provides extra magnification for examination and laser treatment. (Courtesy of Ocular Instruments.)

36

37

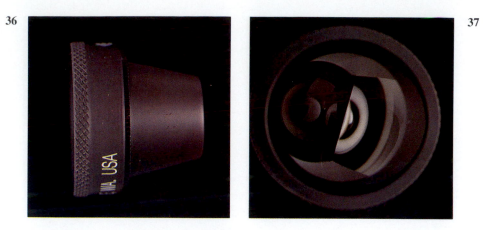

36, 37 The Trokel lens is a Goldmann-like one-mirror lens. It has a broader viewing area than the Goldmann single-mirror lens and a convex anterior face that provides slight magnification. This lens was designed for the delivery of laser energy to the angle. (Courtesy of Ocular Instruments.)

38

39

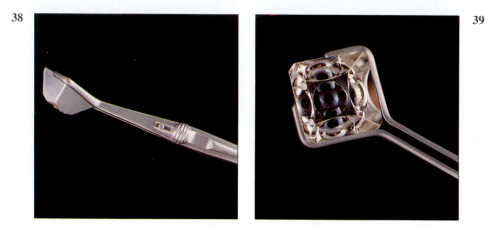

38, 39 Zeiss four-mirror lens on Unger fork. This lens has four identical mirrors for rapid gonioscopy. No methylcellulose coupling solution is required. The small area of contact allows for indentation gonioscopy. (Carl Zeiss.)

mirrors are directed at the angle; two mirrors face the angle at 59° and the other pair approaches it at 64°. In front of one of the 59° mirrors and one of the 64° mirrors are convex buttons that increase magnification ×1.4 and concentrate laser energy (Ritch, 1985). The Trokel lens (**36** and **37**) is a single-mirror lens that is similar to the Goldmann one-mirror lens except that it has a wider field and provides ×1.1 magnification. It

was designed for the delivery of laser energy to the angle.

The Zeiss lens (**38** and **39**) has four identical mirrors that permit examination of four quadrants with no rotation of the lens (**40**). By turning the lens through only 11° the small areas between the mirrors can be brought into view. Because the lens has a small (9 mm) area of contact with the cornea, the angle can be deepened by pushing on

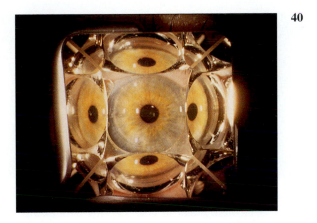

40 Four quadrants visible through Zeiss four-mirror lens.

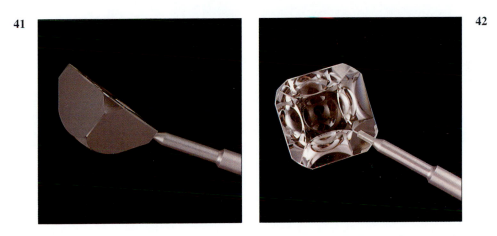

41, 42 Posner four-mirror lens with fixed handle and plastic lens. This lens is very similar to the Zeiss four-mirror lens. (Courtesy of Ocular Instruments.)

the lens. The small gap between lens and cornea is filled with tears or topical anesthetic. This keeps the cornea free of viscous fluids and permits clear examination and photography of the optic nerve head following gonioscopy.

The Posner lens (**41** and **42**) is similar to the Zeiss lens but is made of plastic instead of glass and also has a fixed, rather than a detachable, handle. The Sussman lens (**43** and **44**) is also sim-

ilar to the Zeiss lens, except that it has no handle.

Special mention should be made of the Allen–Thorpe gonioprism (**45** and **46**), which was used in preparing all of the paintings reproduced in this Atlas (Allen *et al.*, 1954). Rather than mirrors, this lens has four prisms. It has a flange that holds it in place (**47**) and requires methylcellulose to couple it to the cornea. The lens is no longer commercially available.

43

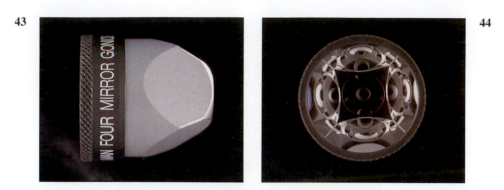

44

43, 44 The Sussman four-mirror lens is like the Zeiss or Posner lens but without a handle. Some examiners prefer to hold the lens directly. (Courtesy of Ocular Instruments.)

45

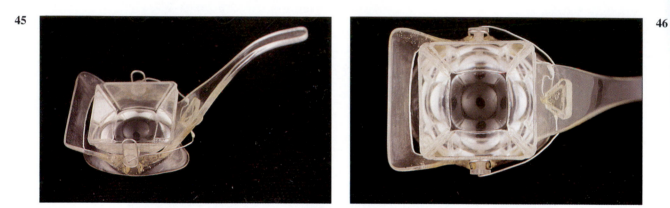

46

45, 46 Allen–Thorpe gonioprism. Four prisms permit all four quadrants to be examined. The lens is suspended in a frame by means of a fine spring that holds the prism against the cornea. The frame holds the lens between the lids. (Bausch & Lomb.)

47

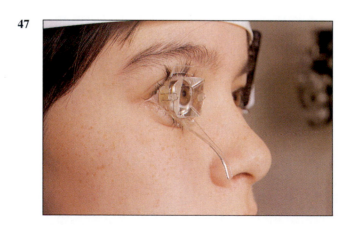

47 The Allen–Thorpe gonioprism is held in place by its frame. Both hands are free to manipulate the slit lamp.

Comparison of Direct and Indirect Gonioscopy

Both direct and indirect gonioscopy have advantages and disadvantages.

Although direct gonioscopy is no longer widely practiced, it does have certain advantages over indirect gonioscopy. Direct gonioscopy, as the term suggests, provides a straight-on view of the angle rather than the mirror image given by the indirect lenses. Direct gonioscopy permits the examiner to vary the angle of visualization more readily – to enable him to look over the curvature of iris bombé, for example. The view with direct gonioscopy is more panoramic than with indirect gonioscopy. Two Koeppe lenses may be used to compare the angles of the two eyes in order to determine whether one eye has suffered a traumatic recession.

The major disadvantage of the Koeppe lens is its inconvenience. The patient has to lie down, usually in a special room with special equipment. The inconvenience of direct gonioscopy led to the development of the van Herick system of estimating the depth of the anterior chamber based on examination by slit lamp. Van Herick stated that 'In the routine examination of non-glaucomatous patients it is impractical to perform gonioscopy' (van Herick *et al.*, 1969).

Indirect lenses have several advantages that have made them the preferred lenses for most ophthalmologists. The main advantage of such lenses is their convenience. This is especially true of four-mirror lenses, which do not require viscous coupling agents. Gonioscopy can be performed quickly with the same anesthetic as that used for tonometry. No special equipment is required. The slit lamp serves as a source of variable magnification and illumination. The slit beam can create a corneal wedge to help to define the structures of the angle (Chapter 4). Indentation gonioscopy can be performed with the Zeiss lens to distinguish appositional from synechial angle closure (Chapter 4).

Indirect lenses have the disadvantage of giving a mirror-image view of the angle, which can initially be somewhat confusing. It is also easy to open or close the angle inadvertently by applying excessive pressure to the indirect lenses. These lenses may exaggerate the degree of angle narrowing and are less able to provide a view into the depths of a narrow angle (Shaffer, 1962). The four-mirror lens is somewhat more difficult to learn to use than the other lenses but, once mastered, is extremely convenient.

Although direct gonioscopy provided much of our early understanding of the angle, an informal poll revealed that few ophthalmologists continue to use this method of examination. The vast majority rely on indirect techniques (Palmberg, 1989). Almost all students of gonioscopy learn with indirect lenses. This textbook therefore concentrates on slit-lamp (indirect) gonioscopy. Further information on direct gonioscopy can be found in the works of Troncoso (1947), Shaffer (1962), Becker (1972), and Kimura (1974). Although these excellent reference texts are no longer in print, they are available in many medical libraries.

4 Techniques of Slit-Lamp Gonioscopy

General Guidelines

The eye should be examined carefully with the slit lamp before beginning gonioscopy. One might see a prominent Schwalbe's line, atrophy of the iris, or evidence of previous inflammation, surgery or trauma. Such findings can provide valuable information that will guide the gonioscopic examination. Tonometry should be performed before gonioscopy; excessive pressure on the eye can artificially lower the intraocular pressure.

The eye should be anesthetized with a topical agent such as proparacaine. Seat the patient comfortably at the slit lamp with the head pressed firmly against the headband (**48**). It is important that both the patient and the examiner be comfortable and braced. Align the lateral canthus of the patient's eye with the canthal marker of the slit lamp (**48**). This will permit sufficient vertical excursion of the slit lamp to enable the superior and inferior mirrors to be viewed. The examiner's elbow should rest on the slit-lamp table or a support (**49**). The magnification of the slit lamp should be set at ×10–25. A fairly short and narrow beam of light is preferred: if the light enters the pupil it will cause pupillary constriction and may make a narrow angle appear more open. A beam that is 2–3 mm long works well.

It is most important to put the patient at ease during gonioscopy. This becomes much easier with experience – that of the examiner as well as that of the patient. If the examiner moves smoothly and with a minimum of drama the examination will not be unpleasant for either party.

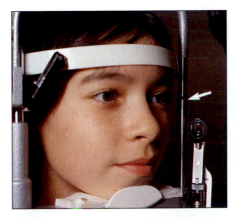

48 The patient's head should be braced firmly against the headband of the slit lamp. The lateral canthus of the eye is lined up with the canthal marker of the slit lamp (arrow).

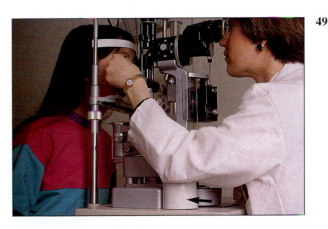

49 The examiner's elbow must be well supported. For examiners with short arms an elbow rest (arrow) is helpful.

Goldmann and Similar Lenses

The Goldmann one-mirror lens, the Goldmann three-mirror lens, the Ritch lens, and the Trokel lens are all handled in a similar manner. All have mirrors that are directed at the angle. In addition to the gonioscopic mirror, the Goldmann three-mirror lens has two mirrors through which the peripheral retina can be viewed. As with all slit-lamp goniolenses, the central optic can be used to examine the posterior pole of the fundus. The Goldmann lens provides an outstanding view of the optic disc and fundus.

The concave face of the Goldmann lens should be filled with a methylcellulose coupling fluid before it is applied to the eye. Care should be taken to keep air bubbles out of the solution. Any air bubbles can seriously interfere with examination and photography. Although some small bubbles can be squeezed out of the fluid or viewed around, they are best avoided. This can be accomplished in a number of ways. The methylcellulose bottle should be stored upside down. If a slow stream of methylcellulose is first squeezed from the bottle on to a tissue, any air trapped in the tip of the bottle will escape (**50**). The stream is then transferred to the Goldmann lens (**51**). Alter-

natively, some examiners remove the top of the dropper to avoid squeezing air into the lens (**52**).

While the patient is looking up the inferior edge of the Goldmann lens is brought into contact with the inferior sclera (**53**). As the patient looks straight ahead the lens is tilted forward over the cornea (**54**). A seal forms when the lens is pressed forward, helping to hold it in place. The examination is carried out through the shortest mirror of the three-mirror lens.

Holding the lens with three fingers of one hand, the examiner can rotate the lens easily, leaving the other hand free to operate the slit lamp. The thumb, index, and middle finger are used to hold the lens and the other two fingers are braced against the patient's cheek to enable the examiner to keep up with small movements of the head (**55**). The lens should be held lightly. Excessive pressure can cause reflux of blood into Schlemm's canal. The suction created by pulling on the lens may make the angle appear artificially deep.

Sometimes, these lenses are difficult to remove because a tight seal has formed between the lens and the eye. Gentle pressure with the index finger on the globe next to the lens will break the seal.

50

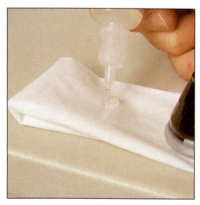

51

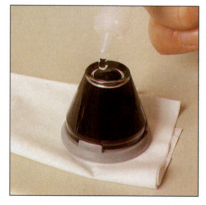

52

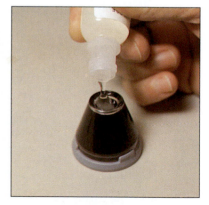

50 Begin stream of methylcellulose on to tissue to release the small amount of air that becomes trapped in the tip of the bottle.

51 Maintain pressure on the bottle to keep air from refluxing into the bottle and transfer the stream of methylcellulose to the lens.

52 With the tip removed from the bottle methylcellulose can be poured without bubbles forming.

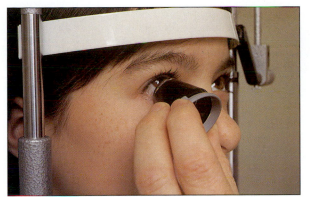

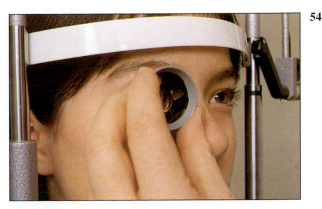

53 The Goldmann lens is brought into contact with the inferior sclera.

54 Goldmann lens tipped up into position.

Four-Mirror Lenses

The Zeiss, Posner, and Sussman lenses are normally used with only the tear film coupling them optically to the cornea. Occasionally, a drop of topical anesthetic or saline in the concavity of the lens will make the contact easier. The lens is generally used on a handle that is held between the thumb and forefinger with the remaining three fingers braced against the patient's face (**56**). The lens is usually held squarely to the eye, which is the most comfortable position for both examiner and patient (**56**). Examiners with long arms may prefer to hold the lens in a diamond orientation (**57**) or to use the Sussman lens. The corners of the four-mirror lens can irritate the eyelids when the lens is held in the diamond configuration. The lens should be applied lightly, just until the air disappears from the corneal interface. The appearance of folds in Descemet's membrane is an indication that too much pressure is being applied (*see* **76**).

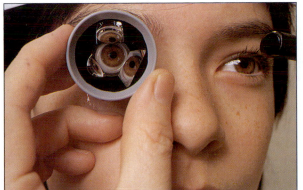

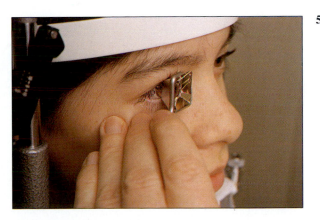

55 Goldmann lens held with three fingers. The remaining two fingers are braced against the patient's face. The other hand is free to control the slit lamp.

56 Zeiss four-mirror lens held between thumb and index finger. The remaining three fingers are used to brace against the patient's face. The lens is held squarely to the eye.

57

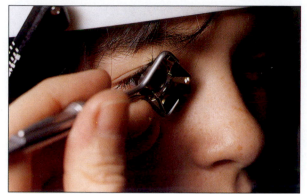

57 Zeiss four-mirror lens held in a diamond configuration. This position is more natural for some examiners, but the corners of the lens against the patient's eyelids can feel uncomfortable.

The View

Slit-lamp gonioscopy is performed through a mirror. The part of the angle that is viewed is 180° away from the mirror that is being used. The examiner must remember that the image is a mirror image. The view, unlike that seen with indirect ophthalmoscopy, is not an inverted mirror image. In slit-lamp gonioscopy the angle seen in the superior part of the temporal mirror is the superior part of the nasal angle.

Variable illumination is an advantage of slit-lamp gonioscopy. One can use diffuse illumination (**58**), focal illumination with a broad beam (**59**), and focal illumination with a narrow beam (**60**). It is helpful to vary the type of illumination and the orientation of the light. Subtle findings can best be appreciated in this manner. Note that in **58** to **60** the switch from a diffuse beam to a slit beam brought the solitary iris process into view and allowed the corneal wedge (as described below) to be seen.

58

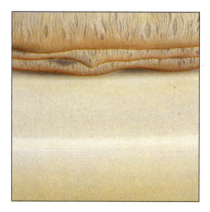

59

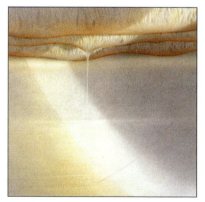

60

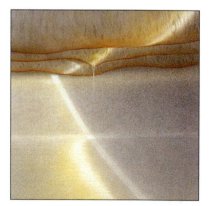

58 Superior angle viewed with the slit-lamp beam fully open.

59 Same angle as shown in **58** but with the slit-lamp beam narrowed into a broad beam. The contour of the iris becomes more defined. Note that a solitary iris process is now appreciated.

60 Same angle as shown in **58** and **59**. With narrow-beam focal illumination the iris process is seen clearly and the corneal wedge is well visualized.

By using a thin slit of light, inclined from the angle of the oculars, two separate corneal reflections are perceived – one on the inner aspect of the cornea and one on the outer. In addition to the inner and outer cornea, the narrow beam illuminates the interface between the cornea and the face of the opaque sclera (**61**). These reflections form a wedge-shaped line termed the corneal wedge (**62**). The lines of the corneal wedge intersect at Schwalbe's line. By pointing to Schwalbe's line, the corneal wedge locates the anterior border of the trabecular meshwork. This wedge can have a variable appearance, depending on the anatomy of the cornea and sclera (**63–65**) In lightly pigmented angles (**66**) or in angles with a confusing anatomy (**67**) the corneal wedge will locate the trabecular meshwork when no other clear landmarks are present. Although initially a challenge, finding the corneal wedge eventually becomes a natural part of an examination. By gently sliding the gonioscopy lens in the direction of the mirror being used, a better view is gained of the cornea and the corneal wedge.

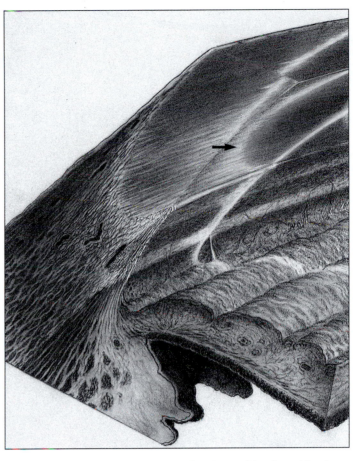

61

61 Drawing showing gonioscopic view in combination with microscopic cross-section. Note the corneal light reflex that is formed as the slit beam illuminates the inner and outer cornea and the interface of clear cornea and opaque sclera. This forms the corneal wedge (arrow).

62 The corneal wedge points to Schwalbe's line – the anterior border of the trabecular meshwork. The corneal wedge in this eye has a rounded contour that reflects the rounded interface between cornea and sclera.

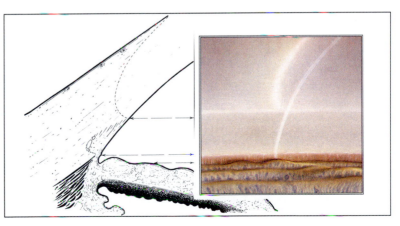

62

63

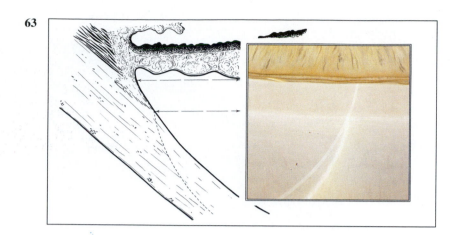

63 Narrow, V-shaped, corneal wedge; this is seen more commonly in the superior angle.

64

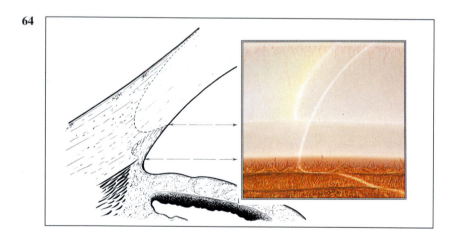

64 Rounded, long corneal wedge, the anterior surface of which disappears behind the trabecular meshwork. The vascular pattern of the corneal margin of the limbus is seen.

65

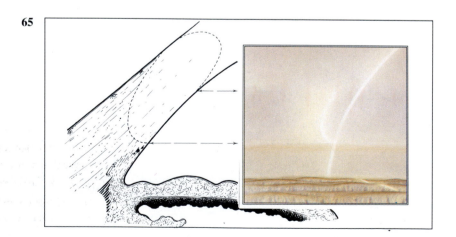

65 Only the tip of the corneal wedge is seen in this view because of an arcus senilis in the upper portion of the view.

66 The corneal wedge points to Schwalbe's line in this lightly pigmented angle of an 11-year-old child.

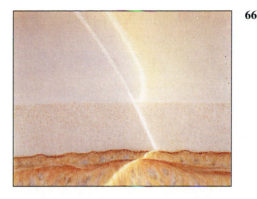

66

67 In this angle the two pigment lines were felt to represent the pigmented trabecular meshwork (line nearest the iris) and a Sampaolesi's line. The corneal wedge reveals that both of these pigment lines are anterior to Schwalbe's line, which is at the level of the iris attachment. Synechiae have caused the trabecular meshwork to be covered by the iris. The pigment lines have arisen from chronic contact of the iris with the cornea or from inflammation.

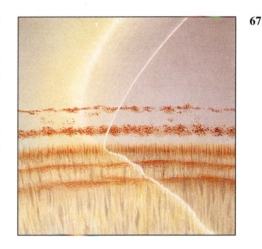

67

The design of the slit lamp is such that the corneal wedge is best identified in the superior or inferior mirror because it is easiest to generate an inclined vertical slit beam in these mirrors. An inclined horizontal slit beam can be obtained in the nasal and temporal mirrors (**68**), but this requires considerable manipulation of the slit lamp. I usually examine the inferior angle first (in the superior mirror of a four-mirror lens). The inferior angle is the easiest to examine because it is the widest and most pigmented. I then proceed clockwise; it is easiest to remember findings by their clock hours if proceeding in a clockwise order. If the corneal wedge is used to identify the structures of the inferior or superior angle, it is usually sufficient to study the nasal and temporal angles with broad illumination (**69**). Once one has become oriented to the patient's anatomy the remainder of the examination is relatively easy.

In patients with convex irides the approach to the angle is steep, which makes examination difficult. The patient should be instructed to look slightly into the examining mirror. This will allow the examiner to look over the iris and into the angle (**70** and **71**). The examiner must not press while the patient's gaze is shifted towards a mirror because this can make the angle appear narrower than it is. Patients using cholinergic drops often have a steep approach to the angle due to pharmacologically induced anterior movement of the lens and iris. If the angle is not capable of closure anti-cholinergic drops can be given to deepen the central chamber and improve the view. This is sometimes helpful in laser trabeculoplasty, although it must be remembered that dilating a glaucomatous eye can cause an increase in intraocular pressure, especially if the patient is using a cholinergic agent such as pilocarpine (Shaw and Lewis, 1986).

Most examiners use gonioscopy to evaluate the trabecular meshwork, but the examination should include attention to the iris and cornea. In the dilated eye the gonioscope can be used to examine the ciliary body.

68

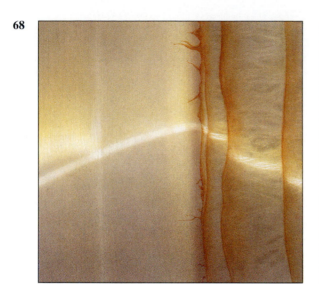

68 The lateral angle viewed with an inclined beam. Obtaining an inclined beam in the lateral mirrors is time-consuming and generally not necessary.

69

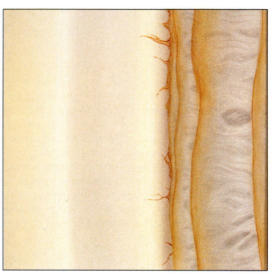

69 Same lateral angle as shown in **68** seen with the slit-lamp beam fully open.

70

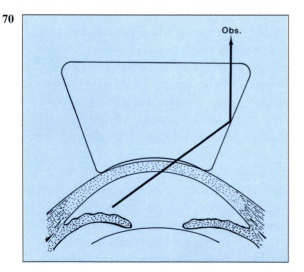

70 Iris bombé makes a direct view of the angle difficult. The forward bowing of the iris blocks the observer's (**Obs.**) view of the angle.

71

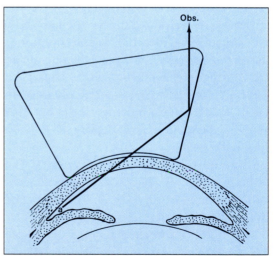

71 If the patient's gaze is turned towards the examining mirror or the lens is shifted towards the angle being examined, it is possible to look over the iris and into the angle (**a**).

Indentation Gonioscopy

In 1966 Forbes described using the Zeiss four-mirror lens to distinguish between angle closure due to synechiae and appositional closure (Forbes, 1966). An eye with appositional angle closure would be expected to do well after surgical iridectomy or laser iridotomy, whereas an eye with extensive synechiae would probably require filtration surgery. Forbes noted that direct pressure on the cornea from the Zeiss lens caused aqueous to be pushed into the angle (**72**). This deepened appositionally closed angles, allowing the examiner to see the trabecular meshwork (**73–76**). Angles closed by synechiae either would not open with indentation or would open only partially, with synechiae tethered to the cornea or trabecular meshwork (**77–80**). For angles that were especially narrow Forbes suggested offsetting the lens a few millimeters in the direction of the mirror being used (away from the area being studied). I find that direct pressure applied perpendicularly to the cornea is a very effective means of opening a narrow angle. Although some distortion is unavoidable in indentation gonioscopy due to the folds in Descemet's membrane (*see* **76**), this does not preclude an adequate view.

At very high intraocular pressures indentation is quite difficult and is minimally effective.

The deepening of the angle as a result of indentation probably arises from a combination of forces. Aqueous is forced into the angle, which pushes the iris to the posterior (Forbes, 1966). The bending of the cornea also results in mechanical rotation of the limbus, which gives the examiner a more direct view of the angle (Palmberg, 1989).

Indentation gonioscopy is effective with such lenses as the Zeiss, Posner, Sussman, and Allen–Thorpe, whose areas of contact are smaller than the cornea. Lenses with large areas of contact, such as the Goldmann and Koeppe lenses, may make the angle shallower with indentation.

Indentation permits the examiner to look deep into the angle recess for iridodialyses, foreign bodies or cyclodialysis clefts. Closure of a cyclodialysis cleft with an argon laser while using indentation gonioscopy has been described in an eye with a shallow chamber (Partamian, 1985).

Once mastered, indentation becomes a natural part of the examination. It affords a dynamic view of the relationship of the iris and the corneoscleral angle.

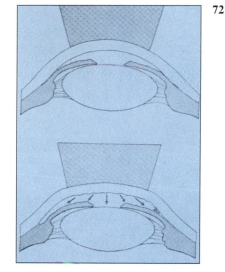

72

72 Indentation with Zeiss four-mirror lens causes deepening of the anterior chamber, which opens areas of appositional angle closure or exposes synechiae. (Max Forbes, MD. Published courtesy of *Arch. Ophthalmol.* 1966; **76**: 488–492. © The American Medical Association, 1966.)

73

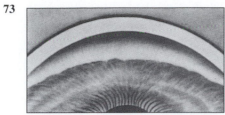

74

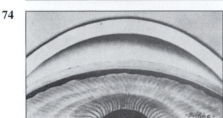

73, 74 Top illustration (**73**) is of gonioscopy without indentation showing angle closure. Bottom illustration (**74**) is of same eye with indentation, showing that the angle closure was appositional. (Max Forbes, MD. Published courtesy of *Arch. Ophthalmol.* 1966; **76:** 488–492. © The American Medical Association, 1966.)

75

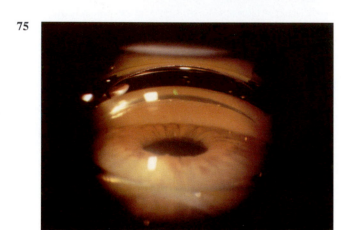

75, 76 The top photograph (**75**) is a Zeiss four-mirror view of iris bombé in an elderly hyperopic patient. The trabecular meshwork is not visualized. The bottom photograph (**76**) is of the patient when a Zeiss lens is used to indent the cornea. The trabecular meshwork is visible (arrow). Note the corneal folds.

76

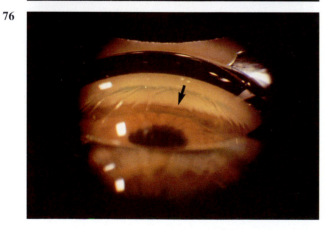

77, 78 Top illustration (**77**) is of gonioscopy without indentation, showing angle closure, Bottom illustration (**78**) is of the same eye with indentation, showing a broad synechia. (Max Forbes, MD. Published courtesy of *Arch. Ophthalmol.* 1966; **76:** 488–492. © The American Medical Association, 1966.)

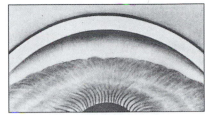

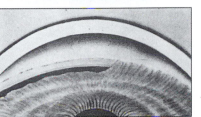

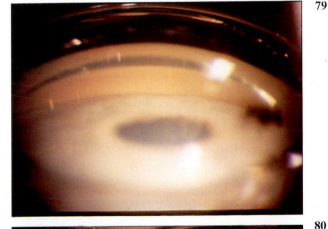

79, 80 The top illustration (**79**) shows an eye with appositional angle closure. No trabecular meshwork is visible. With indentation gonioscopy (**80**) parts of the trabecular meshwork are visualized (small arrow) but there is a broad peripheral anterior synechia (large arrow), which precludes visualization of the remainder of the trabecular meshwork.

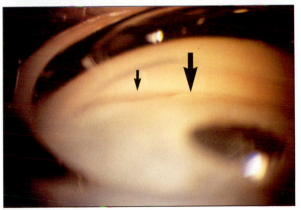

Corneal Edema

When the cornea is too edematous to permit adequate visualization of the angle, topical glycerin can provide some clearing (**81** and **82**). The eye should be topically anesthetized before using glycerin. Even with topical anesthesia glycerin can be uncomfortable. Corneal clearing is rapid.

The examination should be carried out quickly as the effects are short-lived. If visualizing the angle for goniotomy presents a problem, edematous epithelium can be scraped away after wetting the cornea with 70% ethanol.

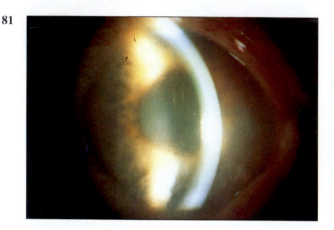

81 Corneal edema precluding gonioscopy.

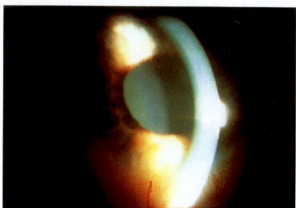

82 Cornea shown in **81** after clearing with topical glycerin.

Cleaning of Gonioscopic Lenses

Human immunodeficiency virus and other infectious agents have been isolated in the epithelium of the eye and in tears. Although transmission of human immunodeficiency virus has not been documented in ophthalmic examinations, it is important to disinfect lenses after each use (American Academy of Ophthalmology, 1989). The human immunodeficiency virus is sensitive to heat and to a variety of commonly used disinfectants such as alcohol, glutaraldehyde, sodium hypochlorite (household bleach), formalin and phenol (Conte, 1986). Unfortunately, many gonioscopic lenses are quite fragile and may be damaged by some of the recommended techniques for disinfection.

In 1988 the American Academy of Ophthalmology, the National Society to Prevent Blindness, and the Contact Lens Association of Ophthalmologists jointly issued guidelines for disinfection. They suggested inverting the contact lens and wiping the surface with an alcohol sponge. For added protection the lens can be inverted and the concave contact area filled with a solution of 1:10 household bleach, which is left for 5 min and then rinsed off with water (American Academy of Ophthalmology, 1989). Some manufacturers recommend soaking lenses in 2% glutaraldehyde or dilute (1:10) household bleach (Ocular Instruments, Bellevue, Washington). Most lenses can be gas-sterilized and some glass lenses can be autoclaved.

With all lenses the manufacturer's instructions for disinfection should be followed to prevent damage to the lens.

5 The Normal Angle

The best preparation for recognizing angle pathology is to become familiar with the many variations of normal. Careful gonioscopic evaluation of the anterior segment follows a routine that evaluates all visible structures in a systematic fashion. This chapter focuses on normal findings, beginning at the iris and moving to the periphery.

Iris

Examination of the iris begins centrally, looking for deposits at the pupillary border that are suggestive of pseudoexfoliation.

Moving peripherally, the contour of the iris is usually found to be flat or slightly convex. Hyperopic eyes have more convex irides, while myopic or aphakic eyes may have slightly concave irides. Abnormal convexity is noted in pupillary block, with large lenses, and with tumors and cysts of the iris and ciliary body. Abnormal concavity is seen in the pigment dispersion syndrome and the iris-retraction syndrome.

The normal iris demonstrates radial markings with crypts (**3** and **83**). Blue irides have more prominent markings and crypts than thick, brown irides. It is valuable to compare these surface features between the two eyes. In some pathologic conditions, such as Fuchs' heterochromic iridocyclitis, the normal markings are lost, giving the iris a flat, featureless appearance.

The iris also has concentric contraction rolls, which are most prominent when the pupil is large and the iris bunched. The most peripheral roll of the iris is frequently more prominent than other contraction rolls (**83**). In some eyes this last roll can obscure visualization of the trabecular meshwork. An abnormally prominent last roll of the iris is a feature of plateau iris syndrome, a form of angle closure that is described in Chapter 8.

The iris should be examined for the presence of nevi, tumors, atrophy, iridodonesis, and abnormal pigmentation.

As the angle is approached the stroma of the iris becomes thinner and smoother. There may be a scalloped border where the iris inserts into the face of the ciliary body.

83 Normal iris with distinct radial markings and crypts. As in many normal angles, the last contraction roll of the iris is prominent but does not obstruct the view of the angle structures.

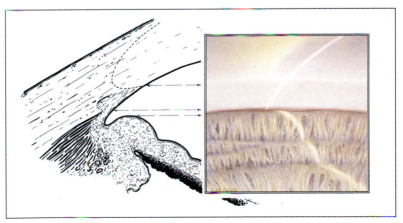

Ciliary Body Band

The iris usually inserts into the concave face of the ciliary body, leaving some of the ciliary body visible anterior to the iris. The ciliary body band is seen as a light gray to dark brown band located just anterior to the iris and posterior to the scleral spur (**84–86**). This band can be quite wide in myopic or aphakic eyes and narrow to absent in hyperopic eyes or eyes with anterior insertions of the iris. If the ciliary body band is abnormally deep and not symmetric with the other eye, the possibility of angle recession, cyclodialysis, or unilateral high myopia must be considered. Both angle recession and cyclodialysis are described in Chapter 9.

84
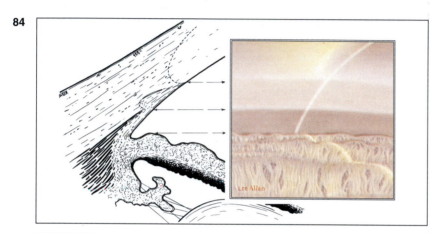

84 Broad, gray ciliary body band, seen most commonly in lightly pigmented eyes.

85
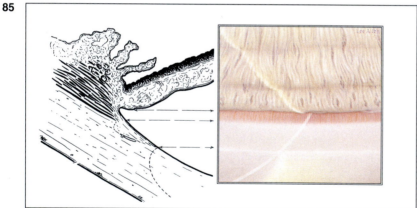

85 Lavender-colored ciliary body band, common with all types of iris pigmentation (superior angle).

86
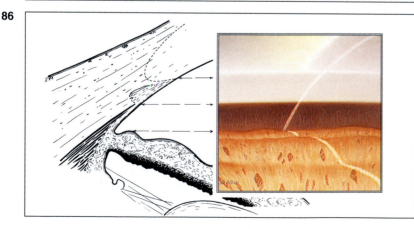

86 Dark brown ciliary body band usually associated with hazel or brown irides.

Scleral Spur

The scleral spur is a ridge of scleral tissue that lies anterior to the ciliary body band and marks the posterior border of the trabecular meshwork. It appears as a thin band that is usually white or light gray (**87**) but which may have a yellowish cast in older individuals (**88**). It may be difficult to distinguish from trabecular meshwork in lightly pigmented eyes except for the striking contrast of the adjacent ciliary body band (**89**). Although the scleral spur is usually visible, it may be obscured by iris processes, a high insertion of the iris, iris bombé, peripheral anterior synechiae, or heavy pigmentation.

87 Narrow, light gray scleral spur accentuated by a low, sharp ridge at the iris root (superior angle).

87

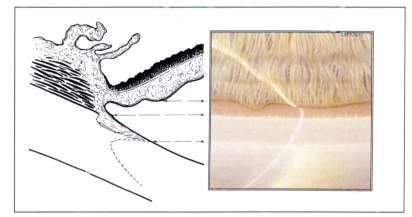

88 Wide, yellowish scleral spur line, an appearance seen more often in the elderly. The major circle of the iris is visible.

88

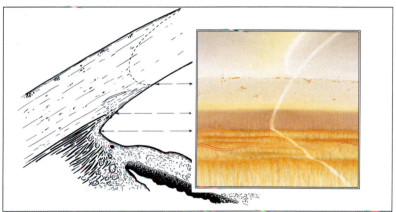

89 Scleral spur of the same color as the trabecular meshwork, identified only by contrast with the color of the ciliary body band.

89

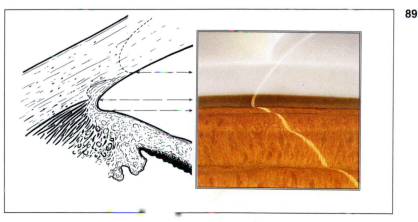

Trabecular Meshwork

The trabecular meshwork lies between the scleral spur and Schwalbe's line. The meshwork is non-pigmented and smooth in infants but becomes coarser and more pigmented with advancing age. Flow through the trabecular meshwork is through the posterior portion. For this reason, the posterior trabecular meshwork is generally more pigmented than the anterior trabecular meshwork. Most of the dark brown or black pigment present in the angle is intracellular, having been ingested through phagocytosis. Skin and hair color show little correlation with trabecular pigmentation (Scheie, 1957). There may be patchy areas of increased pigmentation over the circumference of the pigmented trabecular meshwork.

These are located over aqueous collector channels and represent areas that have more outflow than the less pigmented areas. Patchy pigmentation is seen more frequently in eyes with glaucoma than in normal eyes (Tanchel *et al.*, 1984).

Pigment in the angle is usually heaviest inferiorly owing to gravitational settling and aqueous circulation. With narrow angles there can be more pigment superiorly than inferiorly as a result of apposition of the iris against trabecular meshwork (Desjardins and Parrish, 1985).

A non-pigmented angle is a pale gray color (**90**). Trabecular pigmentation usually appears deep within the posterior trabecular meshwork (**91**). Sometimes pigment is deposited on the surface of

90
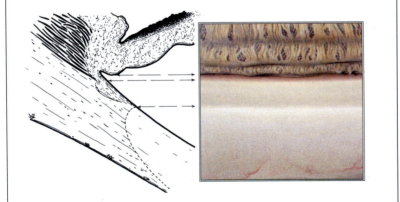

90 Narrow trabecular band of normal gray color (superior angle).

91
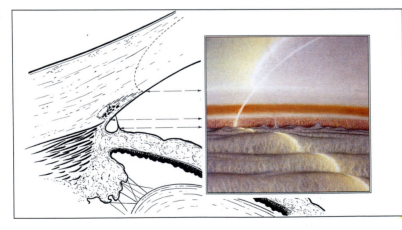

91 Deep pigment in the trabecular meshwork near Schlemm's canal forming a smooth, brown band. A solitary iris process is present.

the posterior trabecular meshwork (**92**) or over the anterior trabecular meshwork and Schwalbe's line (**93**). Heavy pigmentation may cover all angle structures (**94** and **95**). Increased pigmentation of the angle can be caused by many pathological processes; these are discussed in detail in Chapter 9. Heavy angle pigment can accumulate in a line anterior to Schwalbe's line as a Sampaolesi's line.

92 Discrete pigment on the surface of the trabecular meshwork overlying Schlemm's canal.

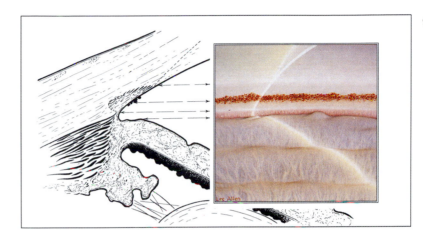

92

93 Discrete pigment along the anterior margin of the trabecular meshwork with a few flecks anterior to Schwalbe's line (identified by the corneal wedge).

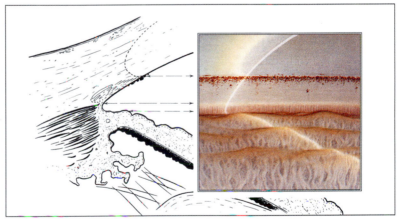

93

94 Heavy angle pigmentation with a wavy band of pigment on the corneal endothelium anterior to Schwalbe's line (Sampaolesi's line).

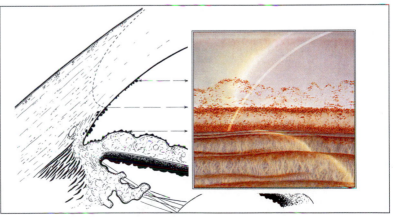

94

Sampaolesi's line is a non-specific finding in heavily pigmented angles, whether physiologic or pathologic. The extra line of pigment can cause confusion in determining the location of the pigmented trabecular meshwork. The corneal wedge can help in locating Schwalbe's line and in defining whether the pigmentation is in the trabecular meshwork or anterior to it. Systems for grading angle pigmentation are discussed in Chapter 6.

The anterior border of the trabecular meshwork is usually smooth, but it can be wavy and irregular (**96**).

95
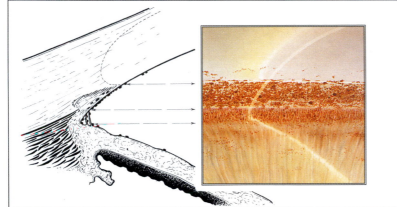

95 Heavier pigment than that seen in **94**. The pigment obscures much of the angle anatomy and is dusted on the surface of the iris.

96
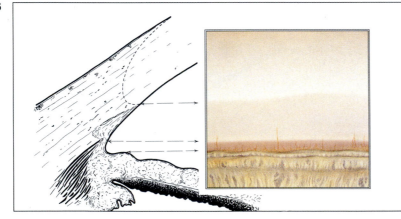

96 Irregularly wavy anterior border of the trabecular meshwork. Note the normal iris processes.

Schlemm's Canal

In most individuals Schlemm's canal is not visible. It lies deep within the posterior (pigmented) trabecular meshwork, anterior to the scleral spur, and becomes visible only when filled with blood (**97**). Blood can occasionally be found in Schlemm's canal in normal eyes. It may also be seen in situations where the flow of aqueous humor from Schlemm's canal to the episcleral venous system is impeded. This can occur when a contact lens with a large diameter (such as a Goldmann lens) is pressed too firmly against the eye, compressing the episcleral veins. It can also be seen when the pressure in the episcleral venous system is high or when the intraocular pressure is low. Pathologic causes of blood in Schlemm's canal are discussed in Chapter 9.

97 Blood in Schlemm's canal. This can be seen in normal eyes, with increased episcleral venous pressure, in ocular hypotony, and with excessive pressure on the limbus from a large gonioscopic lens. Note that the trabecular band is wide and is darker than the adjacent cornea.

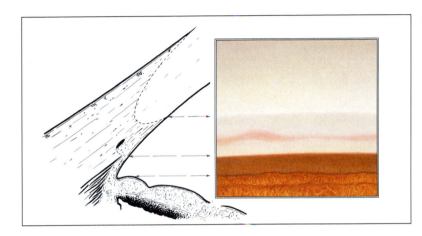

97

Schwalbe's Line

Schwalbe's line represents the anterior border of the trabecular meshwork. It is the termination of Descemet's membrane. Schwalbe's line is usually subtle, marked only by a slight change in color and density from trabecular meshwork to cornea (**98**) and, occasionally, by a faint white line (**99**).

98 Anterior border of the trabecular meshwork marked only by a change of color and density from trabecular meshwork to the corneoscleral limbus. There are scattered iris processes (superior angle).

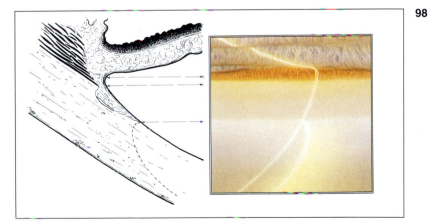

98

The line is often too faint to be identified, particularly in an eye with a very lightly pigmented trabecular meshwork. The corneal wedge, described in Chapter 4, is invaluable in identifying Schwalbe's line. In most eyes the line is a flat transition zone between trabecular and corneal endothelium. In some eyes it forms a ridge-like structure (**100**). When the line is prominent and anterior it is termed posterior embryotoxon. This is usually a normal variant, but it may be associated with the Axenfeld–Rieger syndrome (Chapter 7). Pigment deposited on and anterior to Schwalbe's line is called a Sampaolesi's line, as described above.

99

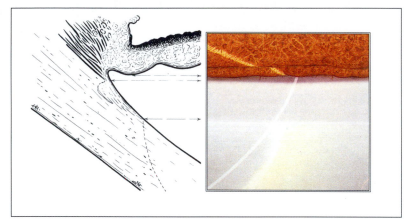

99 Multiple fine, pearly-white lines delineating the anterior border of the trabecular meshwork (superior angle).

100

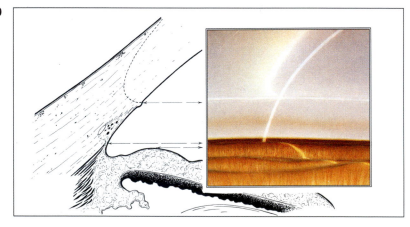

100 Prominent Schwalbe's line forming a ridge. Such elevation is most frequently seen in the inferior quadrant.

Other Regions

The cornea can also be viewed gonioscopically, demonstrating pigment, keratic precipitates, or endothelial changes. Another structure that can be examined in a widely dilated or aniridic eye is the ciliary body.

Iris Processes

Iris processes are often found in normal angles. These are uveal extensions from the iris on to the trabecular meshwork. They generally insert close to the scleral spur but sometimes insert as far anteriorly as Schwalbe's line. Usually delicate and lacy (**101** and **102**), these processes can sometimes be so dense as to obscure the scleral spur. They are abnormally numerous and prominent in Axenfeld–Rieger's syndrome (Chapter 7). Iris processes range in color from light gray (in blue-eyed individuals) to dark brown.

It is important – and occasionally difficult – to distinguish iris processes from peripheral anterior synechiae. Iris processes are usually fine and extend into the posterior portions of the trabecular meshwork. They usually follow the concavity of the angle recess but can bridge the angle. Iris processes do not inhibit the movement of the iris with indentation and they do not interfere with aqueous outflow. Peripheral anterior synechiae tend to be broad and irregular, attaching iris stroma to the trabecular meshwork. They bridge the angle recess, rather than follow it, and they obscure underlying structures. Synechiae inhibit posterior movement of the iris during indentation gonioscopy. They drag normal radial iris vessels with them. There is frequently pigmentation on the cornea anterior to the synechiae caused by the underlying pathology, such as inflammation or angle closure.

With traumatic angle recession iris processes can be broken. This is one subtle sign of recession.

101 Dense band of non-pigmented iris processes bridging the angle.

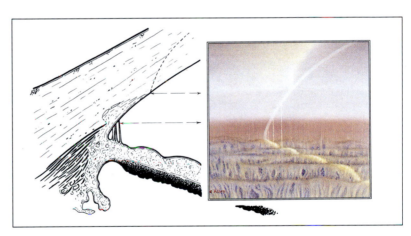

101

102 Heavily pigmented iris processes against the wall of the superior angle.

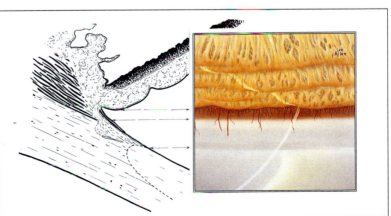

102

Angle Blood Vessels

Typically, normal angle blood vessels have a radial orientation in the iris or form looping branches from the major arterial circle. Although the major circle is usually located in the ciliary muscle, it may occasionally be seen in the periphery of the iris. Short segments of the major circle are often visible in lightly pigmented irides and are sometimes visible in darkly pigmented irides (**103**) (Henkind, 1964). Pathologic angle vessels tend to be fine, cross the scleral spur, and branch. They do not follow any radial or circumferential pattern. Pathologic vessels have associated fibrous tissue, which is not visible.

Angle Width

The angle between the iris and the cornea is usually wide enough to permit a good view of all angle structures (**104**). The angle is generally quite wide in myopic eyes (**105**) and narrower in hyperopic eyes. Angle closure is rare in myopic eyes, although there are exceptions (van Herick *et al.*, 1969). Aphakic and pseudophakic eyes tend to have rather wide angles because of the loss of lens thickness behind the iris.

Many factors determine the width of the angle, including the level of insertion of the iris into the angle, the shape of the iris, pupil size, lens thickness, and the degree of lens–iris apposition.

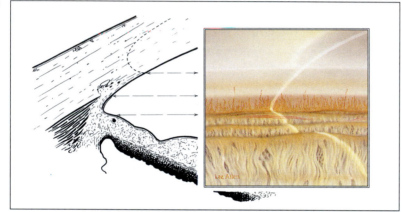

103 Major circle of the iris visible in the angle. This normal structure is usually seen in blue or hazel eyes.

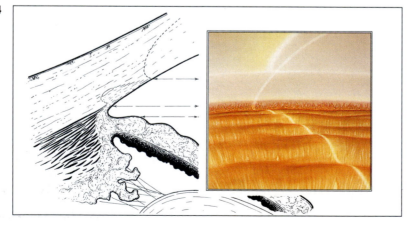

104 Chamber angle of average width. In most eyes the inferior angle is widest, the lateral quadrants are narrower, and the superior angle is narrowest.

Sometimes the iris inserts so far anteriorly that it obscures the ciliary body band, the scleral spur, and even parts of the trabecular meshwork (**106**).

The angle narrows with age. Raeder (1923) attributed this to increasing thickness of the lens. A study of 947 normal subjects showed that the mean age for a closed angle was 85 years, while the mean age for a Shaffer grade IV angle was 25 years (Spaeth, 1971). Van Herick *et al.* (1969) used the slit lamp to examine 2185 individuals. They found that grade I and II angles were present in 6% of those over 60 years of age and in none of those under 20 years of age .

Usually the superior angle is the narrowest, the inferior angle is the widest, and the lateral angles are of intermediate width (Barkan *et al.,* 1936).

Cholinergic stimulating agents, such as pilocarpine, cause the lens–iris diaphragm to move forward. This narrows the angle and makes the approach to the angle steeper. Rarely, cholinergic agents can cause pupillary block and closure of the angle. Angle narrowing caused by cholinergic agents can be reversed by anticholinergic drugs, which tend to widen the angle.

Uneven angle width can be caused by cysts of the iris or ciliary body, angle recession, and cyclodialysis.

Systems for grading the width of the angle are described in Chapter 6.

105 Wide chamber angle resulting from the insertion of the iris root considerably posterior to the scleral spur and from low iris rolls.

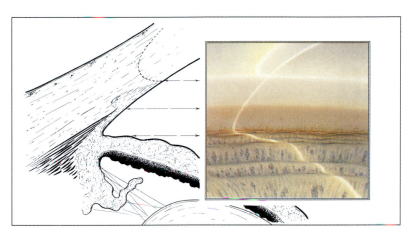

105

106 Iris root anterior to the scleral spur – an uncommon congenital variant.

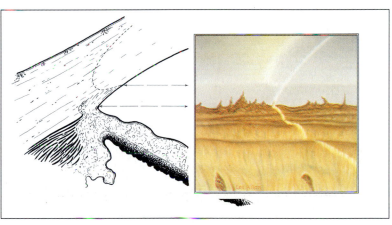

106

6 Gonioscopic Grading Systems

Grading systems permit the recording of gonioscopic findings for communication and for future reference. Several systems for grading the angle have been proposed. Gradle and Sugar (1940) quantified the depth of the angle through a Koeppe lens. They measured the distance from the plane of the iris to Schwalbe's line with a graticule that was etched in the oculars of the microscope. Some grading systems are quite simple – for example the 'wide, intermediate, and narrow' classification of Gorin and Posner (1967). The three primary alphanumeric systems that are currently used for grading the angle are those of Scheie, Shaffer, and Spaeth.

Scheie System

Scheie (1957) developed a grading system in which Roman numerals were used to describe the degree of angle closure. In his system one determines the angle structures that are visible on gonioscopy (**107**). Larger numbers signify a narrower angle. Scheie also described angle pigmentation on a scale from 0 (no pigmentation) to IV (heavy pigmentation) (**108**).

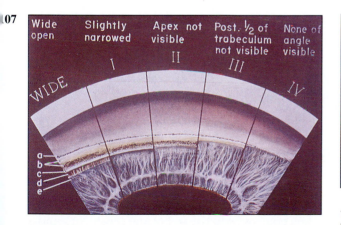

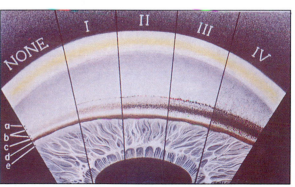

107 The Scheie angle depth system based on visible structures. (**a**, Schwalbe's line; **b**, anterior and posterior trabecular meshwork; **c**, scleral spur; **d**, ciliary body face; **e**, iris root). (Harold G. Scheie, MD. Published courtesy of *Arch. Ophthalmol.* 1957; **58**: 510–512. © The American Medical Association, 1957.)

108 Scheie's system of grading angle pigmentation. Larger numbers represent increasing amounts of pigmentation. Letters **a** through **e** are defined in the legend for **107**. (Harold G. Scheie, MD. Published courtesy of *Arch. Ophthalmol.* 1957; **58**: 510–512. © The American Medical Association, 1957.)

Shaffer System

A more commonly used grading system is that of Shaffer (1960; 1962). This system describes the degree to which the angle is open rather than the degree to which it is closed. Whereas Scheie's grade IV denotes a closed angle, on the Shaffer scale grade 4 refers to a wide-open angle. The Shaffer system approximates the angle at which the iris inserts relative to the trabecular meshwork (**109**). In wide-open anterior chambers the angle between the iris and the meshwork is 20–45°. Angles from 0° to 20° are considered capable of closure (**Table 1**).

Many ophthalmologists use a variation of Shaffer's system in which 4 is wide open and 0 is closed, but the determination is usually a rough estimate of angle width that is not strictly based on degrees.

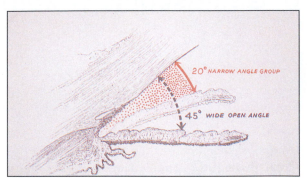

109 Shaffer's grading system is based on the angle between the iris and the trabecular meshwork. For angles of 20° or less angle closure is possible. (Reprinted with permission from Shaffer R. N.: Gonioscopy, Ophthalmoscopy, and Perimetry, *Trans. Am. Acad. Ophthalmol. Otolaryngol.* **XX**: 112–127, 1960.)

Table 1. Shaffer system for grading angle widths.

Grade number	Angle width	Description	Risk of closure
4	45–35°	Wide open	Impossible
3	35–20°	Wide open	Impossible
2	20°	Narrow	Possible
1	≤10°	Extremely narrow	Probable
Slit	Slit	Narrowed to slit	Probable
0	0°	Closed	Closed

Spaeth System

Spaeth considered that available grading systems provided limited information and proposed a system that grades three major features of the angle's anatomy: the level of iris insertion, the width of the angle, and the configuration of the iris (Spaeth, 1971).

The level of iris insertion is represented by letters 'A' through 'E'. If the iris inserts anterior to Schwalbe's line, it is described as grade 'A' (for 'anterior'). If it inserts anterior to the posterior limit of the trabecular meshwork, it is grade 'B' (for 'behind' Schwalbe's line). If insertion is posterior to the scleral spur, the iris is grade 'C' (for the 'c' in sclera). Insertion into the ciliary body face is recorded as grade 'D' (for 'deep') or grade 'E' (for 'extremely' deep) (**110**).

Angular width is the estimated angle between a line tangential to the trabecular meshwork and a line tangential to the surface of the iris about one-third of the way from the periphery. The angle is expressed in degrees (**111**).

The third characteristic that is described is the curvature of the peripheral iris: 'r' for a regular or flat configuration, 's' for a steep curvature

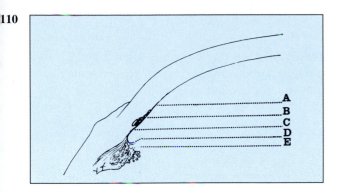

110 Spaeth's classification system includes the level of iris insertion. **A**, anterior to trabecular meshwork; **B**, behind Schwalbe's line; **C**, posterior to scleral spur; **D**, deep, into ciliary body face; **E**, extremely deep. (George L. Spaeth, MD. Published courtesy of *Trans. Ophthalmol. Soc. UK.* 1971; **91**: 709–739.)

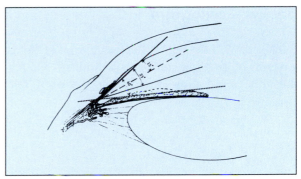

111 In Spaeth's classification the width of the angle is approximated by a line tangential to the iris about one-third of the way from the iris root to the pupil and a line tangential to the face of the trabecular meshwork. (George L. Spaeth, MD. Published courtesy of *Trans. Ophthalmol. Soc. UK.* 1971; **91**: 709–739.)

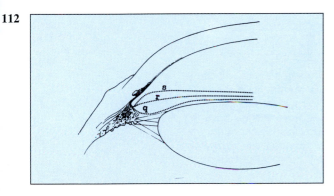

112 Iris configuration in the Spaeth classification. **s**, steep or convex; **r**, regular or flat; **q**, queer or concave. (George L. Spaeth, MD. Published courtesy of *Trans. Ophthalmol. Soc. UK.* 1971; **91**: 709–739.)

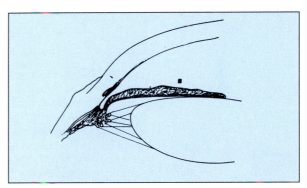

113 A (C)D30S angle in the Spaeth classification. The **D** means that iris insertion is into the ciliary body face, but the **C** means that the steep approach made the insertion appear to be just posterior to the scleral spur until indentation gonioscopy was performed. The number **30** is the angular width of the angle. The letter **S** means that the iris has a steep or convex configuration. This is an angle capable of closure. (Published courtesy of George L. Spaeth, MD. *Perspectives in Ophthalmology* 1977; **1**: 205–214.)

or iris bombé, and 'q' for a 'queer' or concave curvature (**112**).

Spaeth graded posterior pigmented meshwork in the 12 o'clock angle on a scale of 0 to 4+. He also graded the type and number of iris processes.

The Spaeth system permits the inclusion of information obtained by indentation gonioscopy.

If indentation demonstrates that the insertion is a 'D' when it originally appeared to be a 'C', this would be indicated as '(C)D'. Therefore an angle is carefully defined by an alphanumeric description such as (C)D30S – as is illustrated in **113** (Spaeth, 1977).

Becker Goniogram

Becker (1972) described the goniogram (**114**) as a means of drawing gonioscopic findings. He felt that this would allow description of the variable anatomy of an angle within a quadrant. It also provides a convenient way to record synechiae, tumors, foreign bodies, etc.

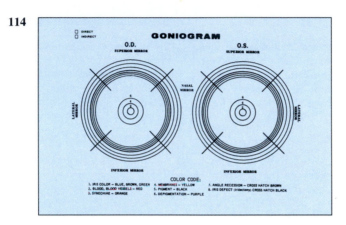

114 Becker's goniogram, on which gonioscopic findings are drawn. The central dark line represents the scleral spur. The three lines outside the dark line represent the trabecular meshwork. The three lines inside the dark line represent the various levels of iris insertion into the ciliary body. A color code is provided for recording findings. (Stanley C. Becker, MD. *Clinical Gonioscopy: A Text and Stereoscopic Atlas*, 1972, p. 79. Published courtesy of The C.V. Mosby Company, St Louis.)

Van Herick System

Mention should be made of the van Herick method of using the slit lamp to estimate the width of the angle (**Table 2**) (van Herick *et al.*, 1969). A narrow slit beam is placed perpendicular to the most peripheral part of the cornea. The oculars are adjusted to give a view at an angle of about 60° from the light beam. The depth of the anterior chamber is graded by comparison to the thickness of the cornea. If the anterior chamber is thicker than the cornea, the angle is a wide-open grade 4 (**115**). If the thickness of visible aqueous is one-quarter of the corneal thickness or less, the angle is dangerously narrow, or 'slit' (**116**).

Van Herick devised the system because routine Koeppe gonioscopy was felt to be impractical; gonioscopy was undertaken only if the angles were thought to be narrowed. Unlike Koeppe gonioscopy, slit-lamp gonioscopy can be rapidly performed on almost any patient and therefore the van Herick estimation is rarely relied upon.

The van Herick test can be helpful in the evaluation of confusing angles because it augments gonioscopic findings by giving a separate indication of the depth of an angle. However, the test does not provide any information about the angle except depth. One could miss tumors, foreign bodies, synechiae, neovascularization, and a host of other pathologies by relying on the van Herick test alone. It is not a substitute for gonioscopy.

115

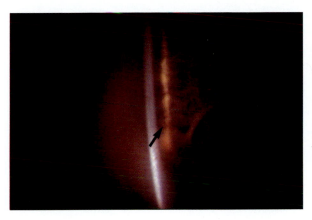

116

115 Angle estimation with the slit lamp by the van Herick method. The beam of the slit lamp is inclined at 60° from the oculars and is placed on the most peripheral cornea. The depth of the anterior chamber is compared to the thickness of the cornea. The depth of this chamber (arrow) is equal to or greater than the corneal thickness and is classified as grade 4.

116 By van Herick testing this angle is narrowed to a slit and the anterior chamber is barely visible between cornea and iris. This is an angle capable of closure.

Table 2. Van Herick system of angle estimation.

Grade of angle	Depth of peripheral chamber
4	≥ corneal thickness
3	1/4 to 1/2 corneal thickness
2	1/4 corneal thickness
1	< 1/4 corneal thickness
Slit	Dangerously narrow

7 Developmental Abnormalities of the Angle

Primary Infantile Glaucoma

Primary infantile glaucoma results from failure of the angle to develop normally. The outflow of aqueous humor through the incompletely developed trabecular meshwork is impaired, resulting in increased intraocular pressure. Unlike the adult eye, the infant eye stretches in response to this elevated pressure. The infant cornea also develops edema at relatively lower pressures than the adult cornea.

The diagnosis of infantile glaucoma is usually made when parents notice photophobia with blepharospasm, tearing, cloudy corneas, or large eyes. Although the disease can present at any time within the first three years of life, symptoms usually develop by the age of three months and the diagnosis is usually made by the end of the child's first year. Most cases of primary infantile glaucoma are bilateral.

On physical examination the eyes are often observed to be large (buphthalmos), with large corneas (**117**). The corneas are edematous (**118**) and may show breaks in Descemet's membrane (Haab's striae), which appear as parallel lines with a horizontal or circumferential orientation (**119**). Gonioscopic examination requires sedation or general anesthesia and is usually performed with a direct goniolens, such as a Koeppe, Hoskins–Barkan, or Swan–Jacobs lens (*see* **18–28**). Gonioscopy is made difficult by the lightly pigmented, amorphous appearance of infant angles and by the corneal edema that is often present in infantile glaucoma.

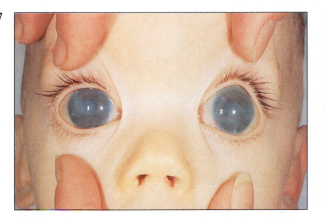

117 Nine-month-old girl with bilateral primary infantile glaucoma. Her horizontal corneal diameters are markedly enlarged at 16 mm. Note the stromal scarring of the corneas.

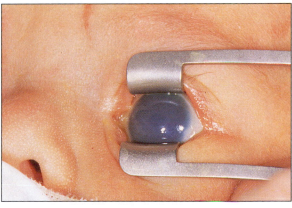

118 Infant with newly diagnosed primary infantile glaucoma demonstrating corneal edema.

The angles in primary infantile glaucoma are immature (**120–122**). They demonstrate a rather flat iris configuration. The periphery of the iris is thin and the deeper pigment epithelium may show through in areas. There is a high, often irregular, insertion of the iris into the angles.

The trabecular meshwork has a generalized sheen due to the thick trabecular beams. This gives the appearance of a membrane, which is referred to as Barkan's membrane – although there is no histologic evidence for such a membrane (Anderson, 1981). The radial blood vessels of the

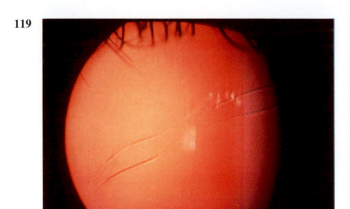

119 Haab's striae in primary infantile glaucoma. These breaks in Descemet's membrane are usually oriented horizontally (as seen here) or circumferentially. Vertical breaks may be seen in obstetrical injuries following forceps deliveries.

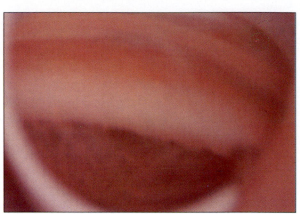

120 Angle of infant with primary infantile glaucoma viewed through a Swan–Jacobs lens. Note the high and irregular insertion of the iris, which covers the scleral spur. There are thin pigmented areas in the peripheral iris. The trabecular meshwork is non-pigmented. (Courtesy of Ronald V. Keech, MD, and Randy Verdick, University of Iowa.)

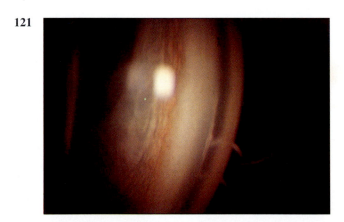

121 Temporal angle of 32-year-old with primary infantile glaucoma. There is a high, scalloped iris insertion and lightly pigmented trabecular meshwork.

iris are often visible and the major arterial circle can often be seen (**123**) (Worst, 1966).

Viewed histopathologically (**124**), the trabecular pillars are thick. The anterior ciliary body and iris insert over the posterior trabecular meshwork. There is histopathological and clinical evidence of traction on the pillars. The traction may cause compaction of the trabecular spaces, with impairment of aqueous outflow. Goniotomy and trabeculotomy cut through the tight pillars and relieve the compaction of the trabecular spaces (Anderson, 1981).

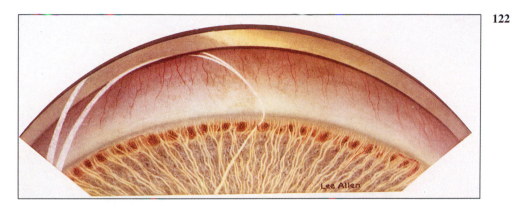

122

122 Fifteen-year-old with primary infantile glaucoma. She was first seen at age six with severe buphthalmos. There is generalized atrophy of the iris with islands of visible pigment epithelium. The iris inserts anterior to the scleral spur. The cornea anterior to the trabecular meshwork is opaque and thin.

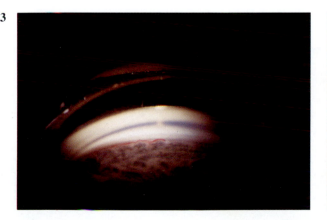

123

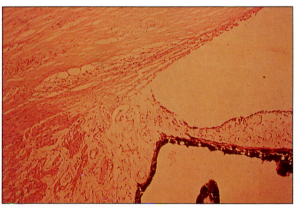

124

123 The angle of a young adult with primary infantile glaucoma. An undulating greater circle of the iris is visible in the angle.

124 Histopathology of primary infantile glaucoma. The iris and anterior ciliary body cover the scleral spur and posterior trabecular meshwork. The intratrabecular spaces are compacted. (Armed Forces Institute of Pathology.)

Posterior Embryotoxon

Posterior embryotoxon is the name given to a prominent and anterior Schwalbe's line. This can be seen on slit-lamp examination and is found in about 10% of the general population (**125**). On gonioscopy Schwalbe's line is observed to be prominent and to protrude into the anterior chamber as a ring (**126**). The ring of tissue may be partial or may extend through 360°. Although it is present in most cases of the Axenfeld–Rieger syndrome, it is usually an isolated finding. Isolated posterior embryotoxon is not associated with an increased risk of glaucoma.

125

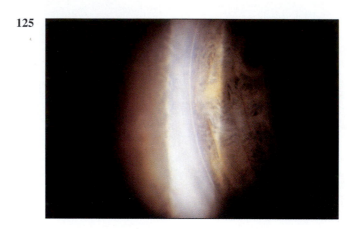

125 Posterior embryotoxon. An anterior and prominent Schwalbe's line is a frequent finding in slit-lamp examination of normal individuals.

126

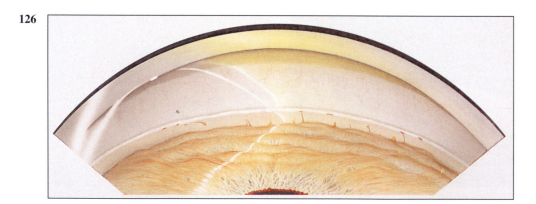

126 Posterior embryotoxon seen gonioscopically as a prominent Schwalbe's line. There are fine iris processes in this eye.

Axenfeld–Rieger Syndrome

The family of disorders known as the Axenfeld–Rieger syndrome includes Axenfeld's anomaly, Rieger's anomaly, and Rieger's syndrome. These are developmental abnormalities that represent a spectrum of anatomic changes ranging from localized ocular abnormalities to systemic abnormalities. Like primary infantile glaucoma, they are developmental disorders of the anterior chamber, but they are morphologically distinct from primary infantile glaucoma. These conditions are usually bilateral and are inherited in an autosomal dominant manner. Glaucoma develops in about 50% of cases, generally in late childhood or early adulthood (Shields *et al.,* 1985).

Axenfeld's anomaly is characterized by posterior embryotoxon with multiple iris processes that extend to Schwalbe's line (**127** and **128**). This line may be dramatically thickened (**129**). It

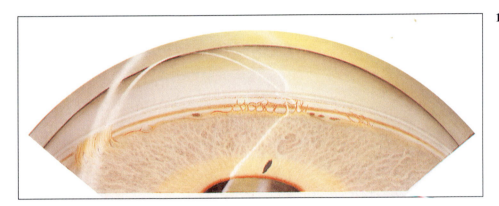

127 Axenfeld's anomaly. Multiple iris processes have formed between the iris and a prominent Schwalbe's line. There is a broad area of iris adhesion to Schwalbe's line on the left of the illustration. (Hermann M. Burian, MD, *et al.* Published courtesy of *Arch. Ophthalmol.* 1955; **53:** 767–782. © The American Medical Association, 1955.)

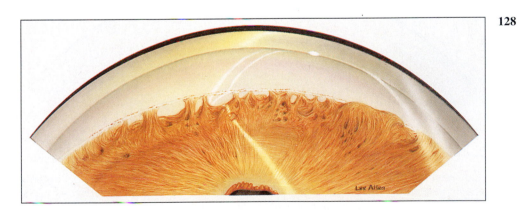

128 Axenfeld's anomaly with dense iris adhesions that almost completely cover the trabecular meshwork. Particles of pigment are deposited along a very prominent Schwalbe's ring. (Hermann M. Burian, MD, *et al.* Published courtesy of *Arch. Ophthalmol.* 1955; **53:** 767–782. © The American Medical Association, 1955.)

may be suspended from the cornea by a fine membrane and can break free from the cornea, leaving portions hanging into the anterior chamber (**130**) (Wolter *et al.,* 1967). The iris processes can be broad or lacy and delicate. The changes to the angle generally affect the entire angle, but they may also be restricted to a small area (**131**). The iris usually inserts anteriorly and obscures the scleral spur.

Rieger's anomaly demonstrates all of the

129

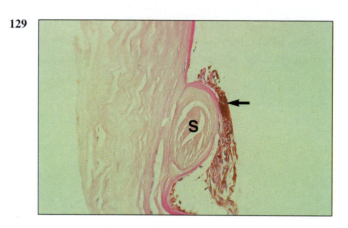

129 Histopathology of Axenfeld–Rieger's anomaly. Note the markedly thickened Schwalbe's line (**S**) with adherent iris process (arrow).

130

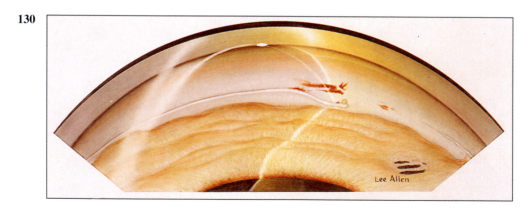

130 Axenfeld's anomaly with partially detached Schwalbe's ring within the anterior chamber. (Hermann M. Burian, MD, *et al.* Published courtesy of *Arch. Ophthalmol.* 1955; **53**: 767–782. © The American Medical Association, 1955.)

changes seen in Axenfeld's anomaly with the addition of abnormalities of the iris. The iris is thinned, with areas of atrophy and hole formation. This leads to polycoria (multiple pupils) (**132**) and corectopia (a displaced pupil)

(**133**). Hole formation generally occurs 180° from the direction of the displaced pupil. Occasionally the changes to the iris can be progressive (Judisch *et al.*, 1979).

In Rieger's syndrome the ocular changes of

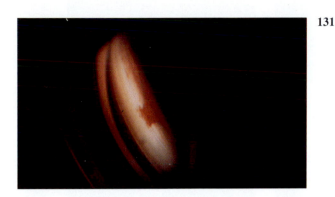

131 The angle of a man examined because his infant son was diagnosed as having bilateral Axenfeld's anomaly with severe secondary glaucoma. The family history is otherwise negative for Axenfeld's anomaly and for glaucoma. This man had one small area of prominent Schwalbe's line with iris adhesions. In other respects both eyes were normal and the intraocular pressures were normal.

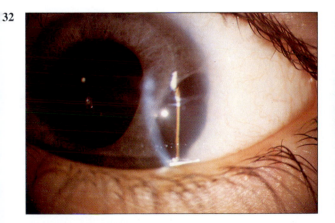

132 Polycoria in Rieger's anomaly.

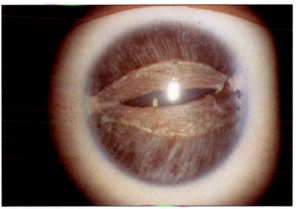

133 Corectopia in Rieger's syndrome. The pupil has been stretched horizontally. The superior and inferior iris are thin. The same patient is shown in **134–136**. (G. Frank Judisch, MD, *et al.* Published courtesy of *Arch. Ophthalmol.* 1979; **97**: 2120–2122. © The American Medical Association, 1979.)

Rieger's anomaly are associated with systemic abnormalities. The most common abnormalities include: maxillary hypoplasia (**134**), small and missing teeth (microdontia and hypodontia) (**135**), redundant periumbilical skin (**136**), and hypospadius.

134

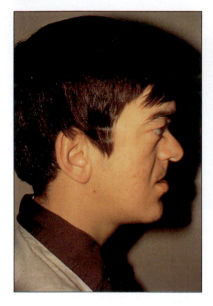

135

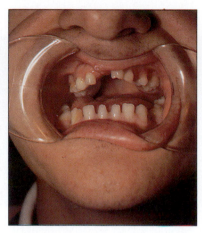

136

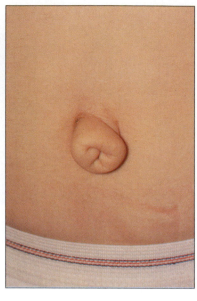

134 Rieger's syndrome, showing poorly developed maxilla with flat face (same patient as in **133, 135** and **136**). (G. Frank Judisch, MD, *et al.* Published courtesy of *Arch. Ophthalmol.* 1979; **97:** 2120–2122. © The American Medical Association, 1979.)

135 Rieger's syndrome showing microdontia and hypodontia (same patient as in **133, 134** and **136**). (G. Frank Judisch, MD, *et al.* Published courtesy of *Arch. Ophthalmol.* 1979; **97:** 2120–2122. © The American Medical Association, 1979.)

136 Redundant periumbilical skin in Rieger's syndrome (same patient as in **133–135**). (G. Frank Judisch, MD, *et al.* Published courtesy of Arch. Ophthalmol. 1979; **97:** 2120– 2122. © The American Medical Association, 1979.)

Aniridia

Although aniridic patients usually appear to have no iris on examination with a slit lamp, some iris tissue is always present. In general the iris stump is so small that it can be seen only gonioscopically (**137** and **138**) or histopathologically (**139**).

Aniridia shows many variations. Most patients also have corneal pannus (**140**), nystagmus, cataract (**141**), foveal hypoplasia (**142**), and poor vision. The disease is usually autosomal dominant but may be autosomal recessive or sporadic. The autosomal recessive form may be associated with mental retardation. The sporadic form may be associated with Wilm's tumor. Some aniridic families have relatively normal visual acuity (Maumenee *et al.*, 1977).

Glaucoma develops in approximately 50% of patients with aniridia, usually in late childhood or early adulthood. The angle is typically open at birth and closes over time. The mechanism of glaucoma development is thought to be rotation of the iris stump over the trabecular meshwork. This may be due to the contraction of strands of iris that extend to the trabecular meshwork from the root of the iris (Grant and Walton, 1974).

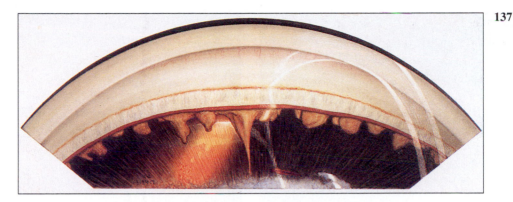

137 Inferior angle in aniridia demonstrating a small iris stump and a pale trabecular meshwork. The eye had undergone a previous cataract extraction. Some opaque lens material remains at the bottom of the illustration. The peripheral fundus is visible.

138 Superior angle in aniridia demonstrating a small stump of iris that covers the scleral spur and part of the posterior trabecular meshwork. The trabecular meshwork has no pigmentation and is identified by the corneal wedge. The patient is aphakic. The peripheral fundus is visible.

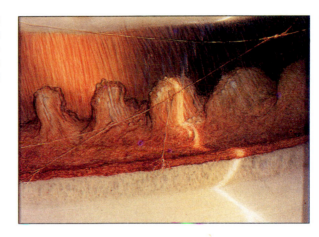

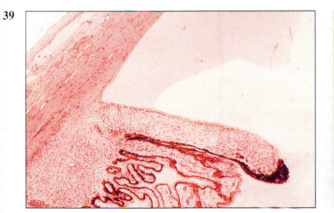

139 Histopathology of aniridia. The iris is very small and barely extends past the ciliary processes. (Armed Forces Institute of Pathology.)

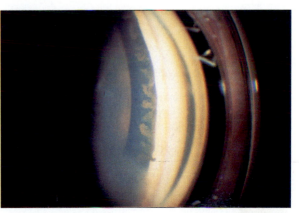

140 Phakic patient with aniridia. Corneal pannus obscures the view of the angle in the inferior portion of the photograph.

141

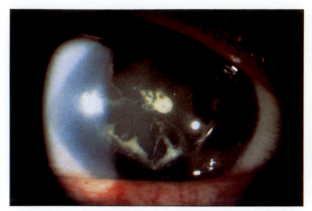

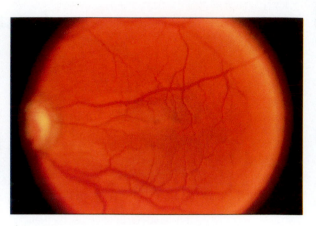

141 Cataract in a patient with aniridia (same patient as in 140).

142 Hypoplastic macula in a patient with aniridia. (Courtesy of Elizabeth A. Hodapp, MD, Bascom Palmer Eye Institute.)

Coloboma

The rare condition of iris coloboma is usually found inferiorly in an eye that is otherwise normal (143). It represents a failure of closure of the embryonic cleft.

143

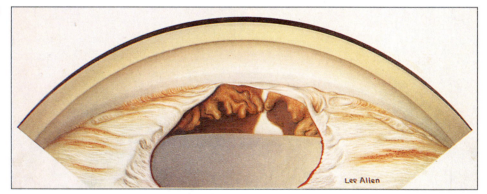

143 Inferior angle demonstrating an iris coloboma. The ciliary body is also absent in this region, allowing the sclera to be seen. The absence of zonules in this region has caused a focal flattening of the lens.

8 Abnormalities Associated with a Closed Angle

Primary Angle Closure

Pupillary block

Pupillary block is the result of abnormal contact between the iris and the lens that prohibits the free flow of aqueous from the posterior chamber to the anterior chamber. Aqueous trapped in the posterior chamber pushes the iris forward (**144**), giving it a convex appearance, which is termed 'iris bombé' (**145**). The outflow of aqueous is impaired when the iris is pushed on to the trabecular meshwork. Hyperopic eyes are at highest risk of angle closure. Such eyes have shallow anterior chambers and small corneas (Tornquist, 1956; 1957). Angle closure is uncommon in myopic eyes. The elderly are more susceptible because the growth of their lenses moves the lens–iris diaphragm forward. Angle closure is especially prevalent among Asians. Pupillary block gives rise to three forms of primary angle

closure: acute angle closure, intermittent angle closure, and chronic angle closure.

Acute angle-closure glaucoma is the most dramatic. On the basis of symptoms it was classified as acute congestive glaucoma until the late 1930s, when Barkan was able to classify it by its mechanism (Barkan, 1938). Patients experience sudden, severe pain with blurred vision and may have nausea and vomiting. Attacks generally occur in dark environments or during periods of intense emotion. Pupillary block is most likely to occur in mid-dilation, when there is greatest lens–iris contact. A patient who does not develop pupillary block when the pupil is fully dilated in the physician's office may develop an attack later in the day when the pupil returns to mid-dilation.

In acute angle-closure glaucoma the affected

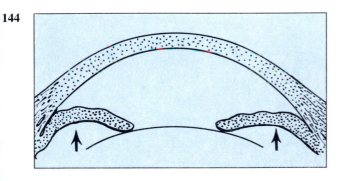

144 Sketch of pupillary block. A relative seal between iris and lens traps aqueous in the posterior chamber. The aqueous pushes the peripheral iris forward, causing iris bombé and eventual angle closure.

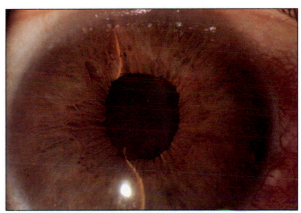

145 Pupillary block with iris bombé. Note that the mid-peripheral iris is bowed forward and that the central anterior chamber is relatively deep.

146

146 Acute angle-closure glaucoma with marked injection and a steamy cornea.

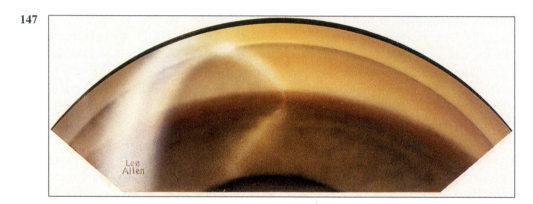

147 Gonioscopic view after an attack of acute angle closure. The cornea is edematous, which limits visualization. The trabecular meshwork has a ruddy appearance.

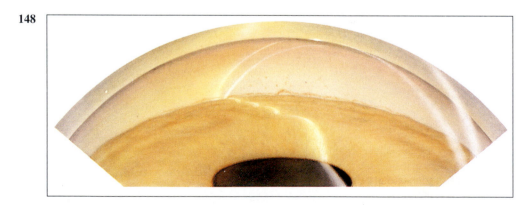

148 Iris bombé. No trabecular structures are visible. Note that the inner and outer lines of the corneal wedge do not meet in the anterior chamber, meaning that Schwalbe's line and the trabecular meshwork are hidden by the iris.

eye is dramatically injected, showing corneal edema and a shallow anterior chamber (**146**). It may be difficult to examine the angle during an acute attack due to corneal haze (**147**). One can attempt to clear the cornea with topical glycerin, as described in Chapter 4. On gonioscopic examination the iris bows forward and obscures the view of angle structures (**148**). Indentation gonioscopy is difficult during an acute attack owing to the high intraocular pressure. The other eye should be examined; in most cases of primary angle closure the contralateral eye will also have a markedly narrowed angle. Although asymmetric angles are unusual, they can be seen in eyes with unilateral mature cataracts, anisometropia, or trauma. If the attack of angle closure breaks spontaneously, there may be an anterior chamber cellular reaction and aqueous hyposecretion. The patient may be diagnosed erroneously as having iritis. Eyes that have undergone previous episodes of angle closure may show evidence on slit-lamp examination of damage from high pressure, such as atrophy of the iris (**149**), cataract (**149**), or spiral changes of the radial iris fibers (**150**). Very high pressures can also cause necrosis of the lens epithelium, which appears as opaque areas (glaukomflecken) beneath the anterior lens capsule (**151**).

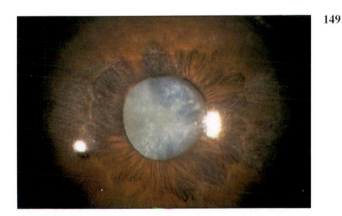

149

149 Dense cataract and patchy iris atrophy in an eye after an attack of acute angle-closure glaucoma.

150

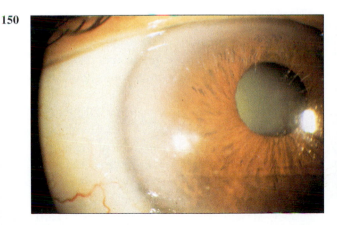

150 Eye after an attack of acute angle closure. Note that some of the iris fibers now take a spiral, rather than radial, course.

151

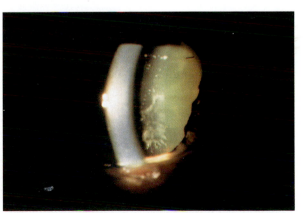

151 Glaukomflecken under the anterior lens capsule after an attack of acute angle closure. These lens changes are caused by necrosis of the lens epithelium.

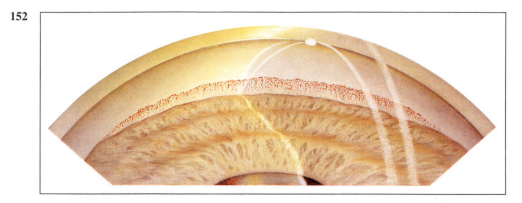

152 Pigment accumulation on the corneal endothelium could be mistaken for trabecular meshwork in this eye with synechial angle closure. The corneal wedge shows that Schwalbe's line and the trabecular meshwork are hidden by the iris.

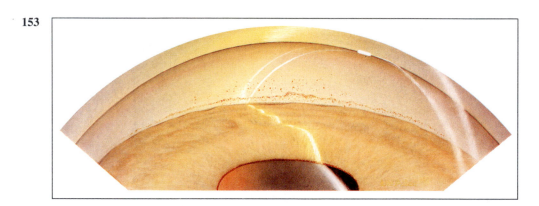

153 Gonioscopic view of an eye with angle closure following surgical iridectomy. This is the same eye as in **148**. There are extensive synechiae and only the most anterior portion of the trabecular meshwork is seen in some areas with the slit-lamp beam.

Intermittent angle closure presents less dramatically. Patients report episodic blurred vision, colored haloes around lights, and headache. Chronic angle closure results in an insidious rise in intraocular pressure without symptoms. In both conditions gonioscopy will reveal iris bombé with very narrow angles (**148**). Trabecular structures may be visible only with indentation (Chapter 4). Synechiae may be present – especially superiorly, where the angle is narrowest. There may be a dusting of pigment on the cornea from contact with the iris, which might cause one to mistake it for the pigmented trabecular meshwork (**152**; *see also* **67**). Indentation gonioscopy

and the corneal wedge are most helpful in determining the true location of the trabecular meshwork. Changes in the optic nerve and visual field may be noted, especially in chronic angle closure.

The treatment of angle closure is surgical iridectomy or laser iridotomy. Medical management is used to temporize and to clear the cornea sufficiently to permit laser iridotomy. Once an iridotomy (or surgical iridectomy) has been performed in an eye with narrow angles the anterior chamber should be noticeably deeper (**153**). Although they deepen, the angles do not usually attain a normal depth; it is unusual to see grade 3 or 4 angles (Shaffer scale) after iridotomy. If angle closure persists after such treatment, the possibility of synechial angle closure or plateau iris syndrome should be considered. Both are discussed later in this chapter.

Unfortunately, some practitioners assume that any markedly elevated intraocular pressure is due to angle closure. They may omit gonioscopic examination and proceed to iridectomy or irido-tomy. It is important to recognize that other processes, such as glaucomatocyclitic crisis, can cause acute and marked pressure elevations. It is also not safe to assume that a marked pressure rise after dilation is due to angle closure. Patients with open angles may show pressure spikes after dilation. These spikes can be quite high, especially in patients with open-angle glaucoma who are taking cholinergic drops (Shaw and Lewis, 1986).

Plateau iris

Plateau iris *configuration* refers to a condition in which the iris exhibits a flat approach to the angle. The iris appears to be on a plane with Schwalbe's line and has a prominent last roll that blocks the view of the angle, especially on dilation. As the angle is approached the iris drops off

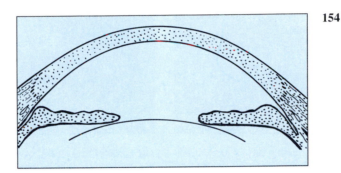

154

154 Sketch of plateau iris configuration. There is a relatively deep central chamber. The iris takes a flat approach towards Schwalbe's line. There is a prominent last roll of the iris before a steep drop-off into the chamber angle.

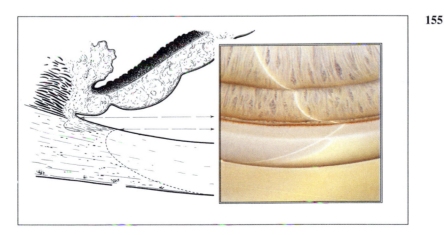

155

155 Gonioscopic view of an eye with a plateau iris configuration. Note the prominent peripheral rolls of the iris and the steep drop-off into the chamber angle.

sharply to insert just below the scleral spur (**154** and **155**). The central anterior chamber is, typically, fairly deep. Patients with plateau iris configuration may develop pupillary block, which can be treated with peripheral iridotomy. If the angle remains compromised, the patient would be diagnosed as having plateau iris syndrome.

Plateau iris *syndrome* is an unusual form of primary angle closure that is not caused by pupillary block. The angle is closed by the prominent last roll of the iris and the abnormal approach of the iris to the angle. A patent peripheral iridectomy or iridotomy must be present for a diagnosis of plateau iris syndrome. In such eyes the ciliary processes are abnormally far forward. After iridotomy the iris is held forward by the ciliary body (Pavlin *et al.*, 1992). On indentation the central iris is pushed back but the peripheral iris is held up by the ciliary processes (**156** and **157**).

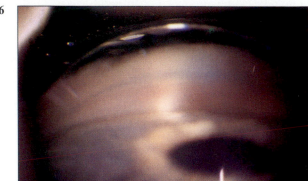

156   Narrow angle in a patient with a patent laser iridotomy. Plateau iris configuration.

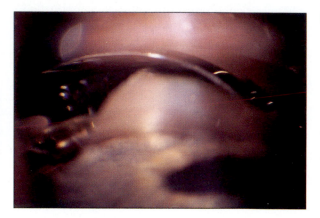

157   Same eye as shown in **156**. When indented, the middle portion of the iris moves back, but the iris over the lens and periphery stays forward. The peripheral iris is held forward by an abnormally anterior ciliary body.

Malignant glaucoma (ciliary block, aqueous misdirection)

Malignant glaucoma is an uncommon form of glaucoma in which aqueous is misdirected into the vitreous cavity, causing the lens and iris to be pushed forward (**158**). The central anterior chamber tends to be very shallow or flat (**159**). Gonioscopy is difficult to perform in malignant glaucoma because of the extreme shallowing of the anterior segment. The mechanism of malignant glaucoma is uncertain. It may be that apposition of the ciliary body to the lens or vitreous body creates a seal that directs aqueous humor posteriorly (Weiss and Shaffer, 1972).

Malignant glaucoma occurs most frequently after intraocular surgery, particularly after filtration surgery in patients with narrow angles. It can occur at an early post-operative stage or later when anticholinergics are discontinued or cholinergics are begun. Malignant glaucoma must be differentiated from other causes of flat chamber with high intraocular pressure. Pupillary block can be difficult to distinguish from malignant glaucoma. In the former the central chamber is usually deeper than the peripheral chamber (**145**), whereas in malignant glaucoma the central chamber is very shallow or flat (**159**). If there is a patent iridectomy or iridotomy, pupillary block can be ruled out; if there is no iridectomy or iridotomy, one should be performed prior to a diagnosis of malignant glaucoma. Suprachoroidal hemorrhage can present with a shallow chamber and high pressure after surgery. Patients with suprachoroidal hemorrhage often give a history of abrupt pain. The choroidal elevation can be seen with the ophthalmoscope or by echography.

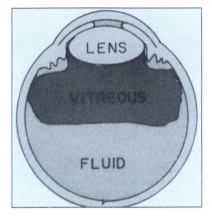

158 Mechanism of malignant glaucoma. Aqueous is diverted into the vitreous cavity and causes vitreous, lens, and iris to be pushed forward, collapsing the anterior chamber. (Richard J. Simmons, MD, Courtesy of *Br. J. Ophthalmol.* 1972; **56:** 263–272.)

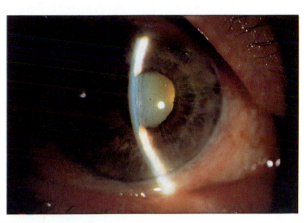

159 An eye with malignant glaucoma following a trabeculectomy. Note that the entire chamber is flat, with lens–cornea contact. This should be contrasted with **145**, which shows a flat peripheral chamber but a relatively deeper central chamber in iris bombé.

Secondary Angle Closure

Secondary angle closure can occur with or without pupillary block. In eyes without pupillary block the iris can be pushed over the trabecular meshwork by a mass or swelling in or behind the iris. The iris can also be pulled over the trabecular meshwork by inflammation, neovascularization, or membranes in the anterior chamber. In eyes without pupillary block peripheral iridectomy or iridotomy is of no benefit.

Secondary pupillary block

Pupillary block can develop secondarily if the iris becomes adherent to the lens or vitreous body or if lens or vitreous becomes trapped within the pupil. Peripheral iridectomy or iridotomy can relieve angle closure in secondary pupillary block.

Central posterior synechiae are inflammatory adhesions of the iris to the anterior lens capsule or face of the vitreous body. If synechiae develop over 360°, the pupil becomes secluded. Aqueous is trapped in the posterior chamber, driving the iris forward (**160** and **161**). Dilation can break the synechiae if they are of recent onset.

A partially dislocated lens can move forward and directly shallow the anterior chamber or cause pupillary block (**162** and **163**). A dislocated lens in the anterior chamber can lead to pupillary block (**164**). In microspherophakia the lens is small and round (**165** and **166**); cholinergic drops induce a paradoxical shallowing of the anterior chamber and an increase in intraocular pressure.

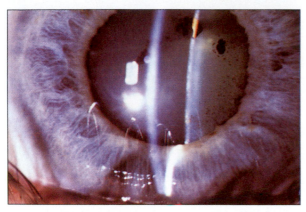

160 Secondary pupillary block due to central posterior synechiae. Inflammatory synechiae have formed over 360°, trapping aqueous in the posterior chamber and leading to iris bombé. (Courtesy of Paul F. Palmberg, MD, Ph.D., Bascom Palmer Eye Institute.)

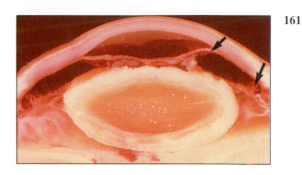

161 Gross photograph of eye with secondary pupillary block and iris bombé. There is adhesion of the iris to the lens capsule, causing aqueous to be trapped in the posterior segment. Broad-based peripheral anterior synechiae are noted (between arrows). (Armed Forces Institute of Pathology.)

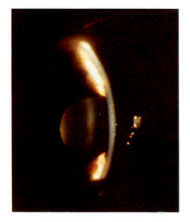

162 The lens is dislocated and has moved forward, causing pupillary block. Note how the iris drapes over the lens, giving a 'volcano' appearance. (Courtesy of Robert Ritch, MD, New York Eye and Ear Infirmary.)

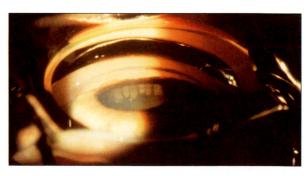

163 Gonioscopic view of eye shown in **162**. The iris is draped across the lens. The anterior position of the lens provides a view of the ciliary processes. (Courtesy of Robert Ritch, MD, New York Eye and Ear Infirmary.)

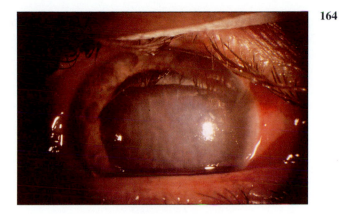

164 Ectopia lentis with the lens dislocated into the anterior chamber. If the lens becomes trapped in the pupillary space, pupillary block glaucoma can develop.

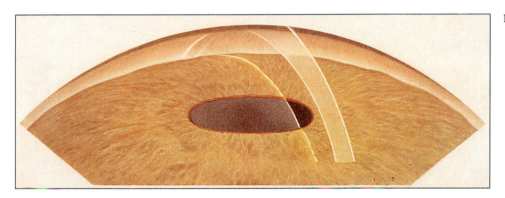

165 Pupillary block secondary to microspherophakia. This patient is an 18-year-old female with progressive myopia and elevated intraocular pressure. Note that the angle is closed and the anterior chamber is very shallow.

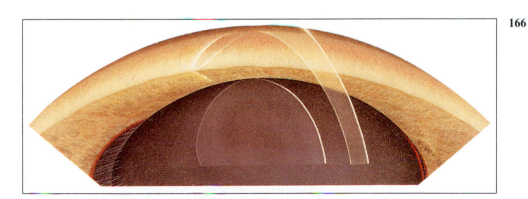

166 Same patient as in **165**. After dilation the anterior chamber is substantially deeper. The trabecular meshwork is still not visible due to 360° of synechiae. Note that the lens is small and round, with the zonules being visualized through the pupil.

This unusual lens morphology can be seen as an isolated condition or may occur with the Weill–Marchesani syndrome. Less commonly, microspherophakia has been seen in Marfan's syndrome or homocysteinuria. Eyes with microspherophakia tend to be myopic and can develop lens subluxation.

Pupillary block can occur in aphakia when vitreous (**167**) or an intraocular lens (**168**) is trapped by the iris.

In phacomorphic glaucoma a mature, intumescent lens can cause pupillary block or can directly compromise the anterior chamber (**169**).

167

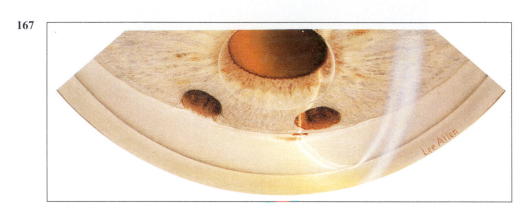

167 Prolapse of vitreous body through pupil. In aphakic patients the vitreous body can prolapse into the pupil, causing a pupillary block unless there are patent peripheral iridectomies, as in this patient.

168

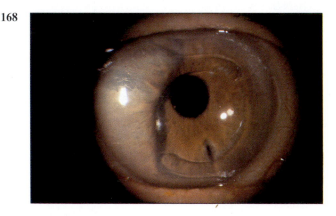

169

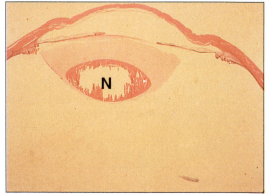

168 Secondary pupillary block due to an anterior chamber intraocular lens. Note ballooning of iris around intraocular lens. There is a patent iridectomy at 5 o'clock, but this is covered by the optic of the intraocular lens.

169 Phacomorphic glaucoma with pupillary block. Morgagnian cataract with a sunken lens nucleus (**N**). (Armed Forces Institute of Pathology.)

Closure of the angle by synechiae

Peripheral anterior synechiae develop when the iris becomes adherent to the ciliary body, trabecular meshwork, or peripheral cornea (**170** and **171**). Synechiae may be small or they can be so extensive that they close the entire angle. They must be distinguished from iris processes. Synechiae are thick and opaque, whereas iris processes are usually delicate and lacy (*see* **101**

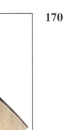

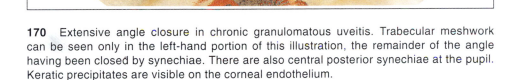

170 Extensive angle closure in chronic granulomatous uveitis. Trabecular meshwork can be seen only in the left-hand portion of this illustration, the remainder of the angle having been closed by synechiae. There are also central posterior synechiae at the pupil. Keratic precipitates are visible on the corneal endothelium.

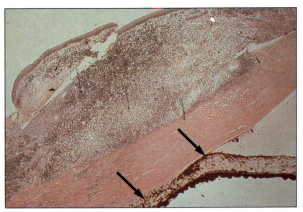

171 Histopathologic view of angle closed by peripheral anterior synechiae (between arrows). There is a large granuloma on the surface of this eye with a syphilitic infection. (Courtesy of Robert Folberg, MD, University of Iowa.)

and **102**). Iris processes are rarely sufficiently numerous to obscure the scleral spur. Synechiae tether the iris to the angle and interfere with the posterior motion of the iris during indentation gonioscopy; iris processes do not. Synechiae bridge the angle recess, while processes tend to follow the recess. The cornea may be pigmented anterior to synechiae (**172**).

Most synechiae attach to the scleral spur or tra-becular meshwork. Although it is unusual for the iris to adhere to the cornea, this does happen in the iridocorneal–endothelial syndromes or after prolonged contact between the two bodies.

When synechiae are of recent origin they can sometimes be broken with the laser or by surgery (goniosynechialysis). Some of the many conditions that can lead to the growth of synechiae are described on the following pages.

172

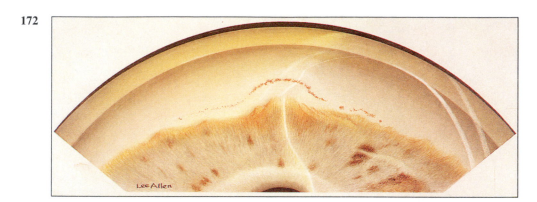

172 Gonioscopic view of eye with peripheral anterior synechiae due to inflammation of unknown etiology. Peripheral anterior synechiae have developed over 360°. Pigment has been deposited anterior to the peripheral anterior synechiae at 6 o'clock.

Neovascularization Blood vessels can be seen in normal angles. The vessels are circumferential at the base of the iris or are radial. Normal vessels do not cross the scleral spur on to the trabecular meshwork. Abnormal vessels can cross the scleral spur (**173**) and may arborize into fine branches that dive into the trabecular meshwork. While the larger branches are seen as small twigs, smaller vessels may appear only as a red blush. Neovascular vessels have an associated membrane that can impair aqueous outflow despite an apparently open angle (**174**). With time this fibrovascular membrane may contract, leading to closure of the angle by synechiae (**175**). Many patients with neovascularization of the anterior segment will first demonstrate new vessels at the pupillary margin (**176**).

Neovascularization can result from many processes. Most cases are due to retinal disease – such as diabetic retinopathy, central retinal vein occlusion, central retinal artery occlusion, retinopathy of prematurity, tumor, chronic retinal detachment, Eale's disease, or sickle cell disease. Ocular ischemia can also cause neovascularization of the anterior chamber. Chronic inflammation can make normal angle vessels become more

173

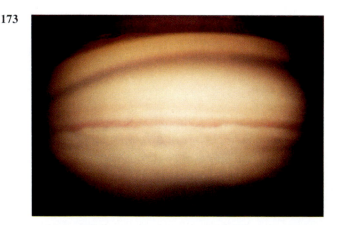

173 Gonioscopic view of eye with early neovascularization of the angle. Twigs of vessels are seen crossing the scleral spur, but the angle is open.

174

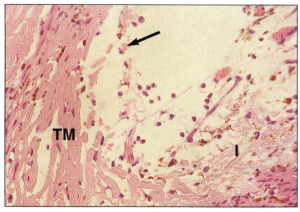

174 Neovascular membrane (arrow) lines an open angle. (**TM**, trabecular meshwork; **I**, iris). (Courtesy of

prominent or can cause true neovascularization. The neovascularization of Fuchs' heterochromic iridocyclitis rarely leads to the development of synechiae. This disease is therefore described under open-angle mechanisms in Chapter 9.

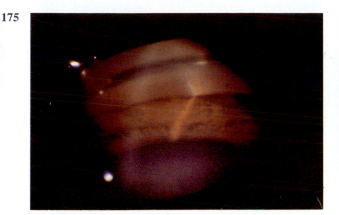

175 Neovascular glaucoma with 360° of peripheral anterior synechiae. Note that the corneal wedge does not join into a single line in the anterior chamber. This finding confirms that the iris is pulled anterior to Schwalbe's line.

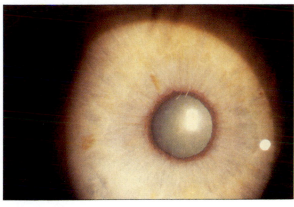

176 Iris of a patient with early neovascularization of the iris (rubeosis iridis). Note the very tiny tufts of vessels around the pupillary margin.

Iridocorneal–endothelial syndromes The iridocorneal–endothelial (ICE) group of diseases have in common changes in the corneal endothelium and the formation of peripheral anterior synechiae. They appear to be the result of an abnormal growth of corneal endothelium throughout the anterior segment. The corneal endothelium demonstrates a characteristic hammered metal appearance on examination by slit lamp (**177**). Specular microscopy reveals markedly abnormal endothelial cells (**178**). The ICE syndromes are unilateral and are most

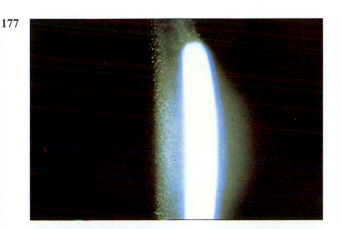

177 Iridocorneal-endothelial syndrome with the typical hammered metal appearance of the corneal endothelium. This patient has Chandler's syndrome.

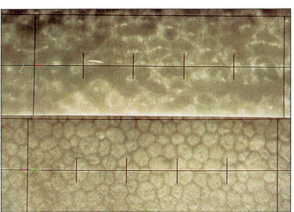

178 Specular microscopy of a patient with Chandler's syndrome (upper portion), showing marked disruption of the endothelial pattern. The endothelium of the patient's normal eye is shown in the lower portion of the figure.

prevalent in women in their 30s and 40s. They frequently cause a secondary angle-closure glaucoma that can be very difficult to treat.

The ICE syndromes are usually divided into three types, but there is substantial overlap. In Chandler's syndrome the corneal changes described above predominate (**177**). There may be corneal edema. Abnormalities of the iris are minimal. In essential iris atrophy the iris changes predominate. The iris demonstrates evidence of melting and membrane contraction. These result in the development of stretch holes and melt holes (polycoria) and a displaced pupil (corectopia) (**179** and **180**). In iris-nevus (Cogan–Reese) syndrome nevi-like elevations develop on the face of the iris; these consist of normal iris protruding through a membrane that coats the iris (**181**).

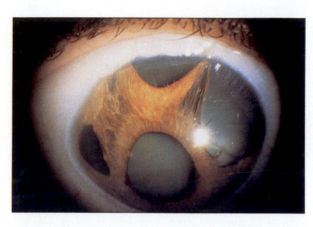

179 Essential iris atrophy showing corectopia with the pupil displaced inferiorly. Also visible are a stretch hole in the upper right part of the figure and a melt hole in the lower left corner of the figure.

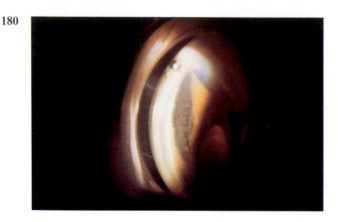

180 Gonioscopic view of eye shown in **179**, demonstrating anterior synechiae with the ciliary body drawn up towards the angle.

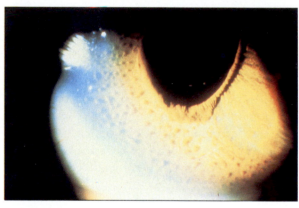

181 Iris-nevus syndrome showing nodular lesions on the surface of the iris. (Courtesy of Elizabeth A. Hodapp, MD, Bascom Palmer Eye Institute.)

Posterior polymorphous dystrophy Posterior polymorphous dystrophy (PPMD) is an uncommon bilateral corneal dystrophy. It is usually an autosomal dominant disease but may be sporadic. PPMD is characterized by the presence of endothelial vesicles (**182**); these may appear in

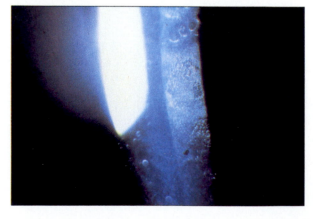

182 Posterior polymorphous dystrophy in a seven-year-old child showing vesicular changes on the corneal endothelium. (Jay H. Krachmer, MD, Courtesy of *Trans. Am. Ophthalmol. Soc.* 1985; **83**: 413–475.)

groups, sometimes with a linear orientation. Often the vesicles are surrounded by a corneal haze. There can be opacification of the posterior cornea. Glaucoma develops in about 14% of cases and is usually due to a membranous overgrowth of the trabecular meshwork (**183**) (Krachmer, 1985). Open angles with high iris insertions have been seen, suggesting a primary angle abnormality (Krachmer, 1985).

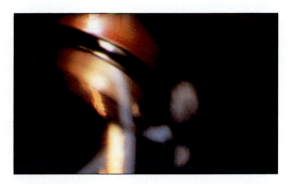

183

183 Gonioscopic view of cornea with posterior polymorphous dystrophy. To the right the angle is open, but to the left there is a broad band of synechiae. (Jay H. Krachmer, MD, Courtesy of *Trans. Am. Ophthalmol. Soc.* 1985; **83**: 413–475.)

After surgery and trauma Flat anterior chambers following surgery can lead to the development of peripheral anterior synechiae (**184**), the location of which may be anterior to Schwalbe's line (**185**).

Epithelial downgrowth is a rare outcome of penetrating trauma or surgery, but may occur particularly when there is inadequate wound apposition. Epithelium seeded into the anterior chamber may form a cyst (**186**) or a sheet of epithelium (**187**). The sheets are clear and can be difficult to identify. Their presence on the iris can be detected by blanching when heated with argon laser energy; normal iris does not demonstrate blanching. As the epithelium coats the inner surfaces of the eye it covers the chamber angle (**188** and **189**), leading to intractable glaucoma.

The synechiae formed by argon laser trabeculoplasty are usually small, conical adhesions of peripheral iris to the posterior meshwork (**190**), but they can be extensive if the laser is aimed far to the posterior and high energy levels are used (**191**) (Rouhiainen *et al.*, 1988).

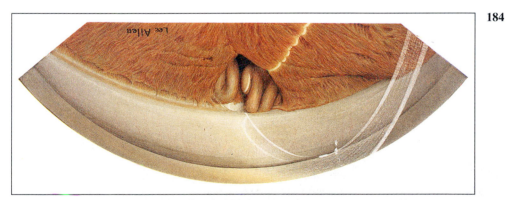

184

184 Formation of synechiae in the superior angle following filtration surgery. Ciliary body processes are incarcerated within the filtration fistula. On the right of the figure is a broad synechia. On the left, the trabecular meshwork is open with scattered low synechiae to the scleral spur. The painting is positioned to show the superior angle viewed through an indirect lens. The artist's name therefore appears upside down.

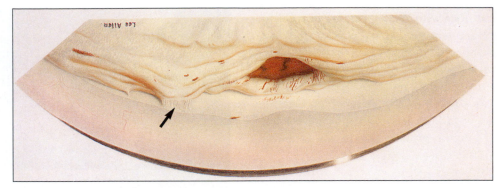

185 Extensive synechiae and iris adherent to wound (arrow) in patient with prolonged flat chamber following extraction of a cataract. No trabecular meshwork is visible. The painting is positioned to show the superior angle viewed through an indirect lens. The artist's name therefore appears upside down.

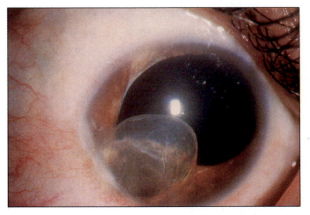

186 Epithelial inclusion cyst in the anterior chamber of a young man who had previously been struck in the eye with a knife. (Bascom Palmer Eye Institute.)

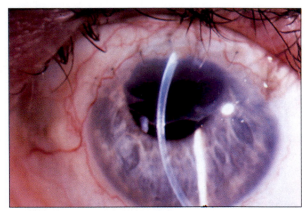

187 Sheet of epithelial downgrowth over the superior portion of the corneal endothelium following extraction of a cataract. (Courtesy of William W. Culbertson, MD, Bascom Palmer Eye Institute.)

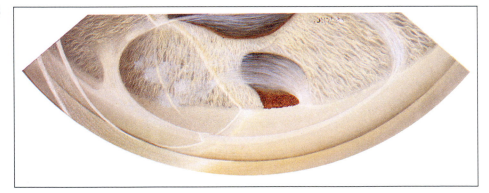

188 Extensive membranes within the anterior chamber causing complete synechiae. This epithelial downgrowth occurred following extraction of a cataract.

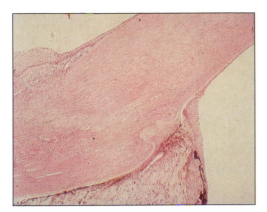

189 Epithelial downgrowth. A multilayered epithelial membrane covers Descemet's membrane and wraps over the iris, which is adherent to the cornea. (Courtesy of Robert Folberg, MD, University of Iowa.)

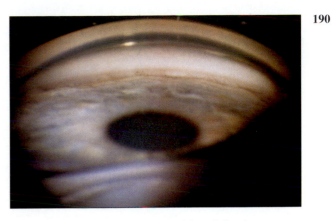

190 Low-lying, tent-like synechiae following argon-laser trabeculoplasty.

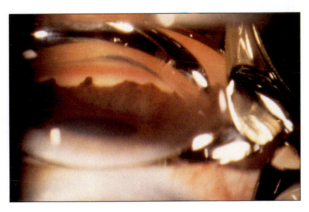

191 Extensive formation of synechiae in a myopic patient who had received laser trabeculoplasty. The energy was delivered very far posteriorly. (Courtesy of Robert Ritch, MD, New York Eye and Ear Infirmary.)

Inflammation Inflammation can lead to the formation of synechiae as consolidation of the inflammatory material in the angle draws the iris over the trabecular meshwork. Synechiae may develop when the iris is apposed to the trabecular meshwork for a prolonged period. If there is both apposition and inflammation, as in a flat chamber following surgery, the tendency for synechiae to form becomes marked.

Posterior pressure

Cysts and tumors in the peripheral iris and ciliary body can lead to closure of segments of the angle (**192**). They do not usually close enough of the angle to result in glaucoma. Some iris cysts can be opened with a laser to relieve compromise of the angle (**193** and **194**). Dislocated lenses can also cause the closure of angle segments.

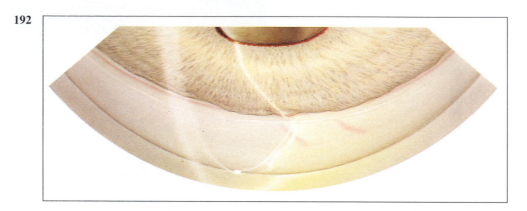

192 Narrowing of segmental angle due to ciliary body melanoma. Note that the iris is pushed forward in the center of the figure and obscures the trabecular meshwork, which is visible both to the right and to the left of this area. This patient has a rather prominent Schwalbe's line and has blood in Schlemm's canal.

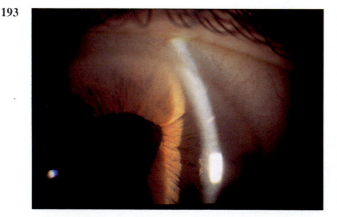

193 Cyst of the iris with segmental angle closure.

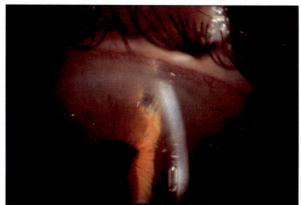

194 Same patient as in **193**, showing deepening of the chamber following laser opening of the iris cyst.

Swelling of the ciliary body

Swelling of the ciliary body can result in angle closure (**195**). Compromise of venous drainage or inflammation of the ciliary body may lead to such swelling. Swelling can also occur after scleral buckling procedures, after extensive pan-retinal photocoagulation and with ciliochoroidal detachment as a result of inflammatory pseudo-tumor (Gass, 1967). Angle closure due to swelling of the ciliary body does not respond to iridectomy or iridotomy. Cholinergic agents can worsen the condition by moving the lens–iris diaphragm forward and breaking down the blood–aqueous barrier. Anticholinergic and steroid therapy along with aqueous suppression is the preferred management.

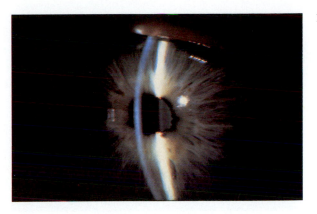

195 Shallow anterior chamber due to swelling of the ciliary body, the result of extensive panretinal photocoagulation.

Iridoschisis

Iridoschisis is a rare iris disorder of the elderly. In this disease there is a bilateral separation of the stroma, especially of the inferior iris. Early in the disease an intact sheet of anterior stroma may split and balloon forward (**196** and **197**). The anterior iris can obstruct the angle. Later the anterior layer of the iris may fragment (**198** and **199**). The fragments may come into contact with the corneal endothelium, leading to localized corneal edema. Glaucoma can arise as a result of angle closure either because of the anterior iris layer covering the trabecular meshwork or as a result of pupillary block (Rodrigues *et al.*, 1983). Open-angle glaucoma can result from the presence of fragments of pigment and iris in the trabecular meshwork.

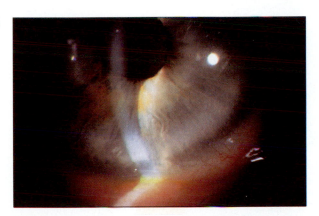

196 Eye of patient with iridoschisis; the anterior and posterior portions of the inferior iris have split, causing the anterior iris to bulge forward and segmentally close the angle (right eye).

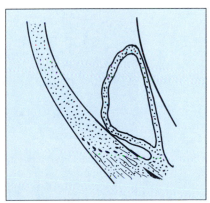

197 Illustration of the process shown in **196**, demonstrating how iridoschisis can cause angle closure.

198

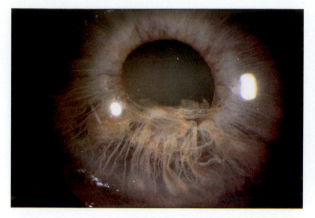

19

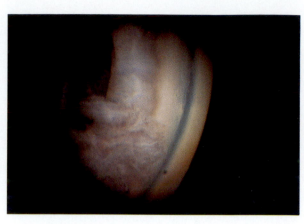

198 Same patient as **196**. The left eye showed fragmentation of the anterior iris. These iris strands were touching the cornea but had not yet caused corneal decompensation.

199 Gonioscopic photograph of eye shown in **198**. Fragments of the iris touch the corneal endothelium in an eye with an open angle.

Fuchs' endothelial dystrophy

Fuchs' endothelial dystrophy is a slowly progressive degeneration of the corneal endothelium. The loss of endothelial function leads to an accumulation of water in the cornea accompanied by an increase in its thickness (**200**). In rare cases the thickening of the cornea can cause angle closure, particularly in an eye with already narrow angles.

200

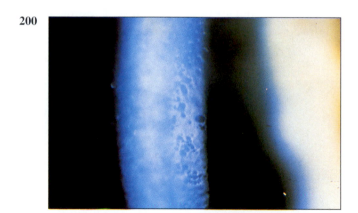

200 Fuchs' endothelial dystrophy. Marked thickening of the cornea with extensive guttata. Rarely, these patients will develop angle closure. (Courtesy of Jay H. Krachmer, MD, University of Minnesota.)

9 Abnormalities Associated with an Open Angle

Primary Open-Angle Glaucoma

Primary open-angle glaucoma is the most prevalent form of glaucoma. It is mentioned here only to note that there are no characteristic gonioscopic abnormalities in primary open-angle glaucoma, ocular hypertension, or normal-tension glaucoma.

Material Deposited in the Angle

Pigment

Pigment dispersion syndrome   In the pigment dispersion syndrome there is an accumulation of pigment on structures throughout the anterior segment. The pigment originates from the iris pigment epithelium, which is abraded against the lens zonules (Campbell, 1979). As the pigment circulates throughout the anterior segment it is deposited at many sites. The syndrome is most common in young myopic individuals. Although the pigment dispersion syndrome is equally prevalent in both sexes, pigmentary glaucoma develops more commonly in males.

With the slit lamp pigment deposited by aqueous convection currents can be seen as a vertical band on the corneal endothelium – the Krukenberg spindle (**201**). The dusting of pigment on the surface of the iris can occasionally be sufficiently dense to cause heterochromia (**202**). Characteristic spoke-like defects of the iris pigment epithelium are seen by transillumination (**203**).

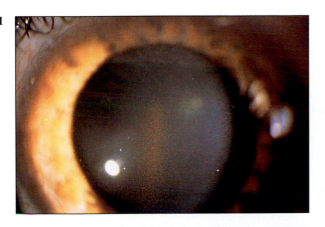

201 Krukenberg spindle in the pigment dispersion syndrome. Pigment released from the pigment epithelium of the posterior iris is deposited by convection currents on the corneal endothelium in a vertical band.

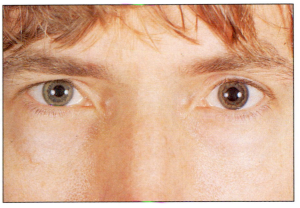

202 Iris heterochromia due to pigment dispersion in the left edge of a patient with the pigment dispersion syndrome. Also note that the left pupil is larger than the right: anisocoria can be seen in the pigment dispersion syndrome, the larger pupil generally being on the side with more transillumination defects. (William L. Haynes, MD; courtesy of *Am. J. Ophthalmol.* 1991; **112**: 463–464.)

Gonioscopic examination reveals dense black pigmentation of the trabecular meshwork and throughout the angle (**204**). Pigment is frequently deposited anterior to Schwalbe's line as a Sampaolesi's line, which is a non-specific sign of increased pigmentation. There may be a concavity of the mid-peripheral iris, which probably contributes to iris–zonule contact (**205**).

203

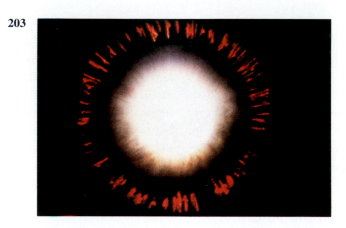

203 Characteristic spoke-like transillumination defects in the iris of a patient with the pigment dispersion syndrome. These defects are caused when the iris pigment epithelium is rubbed off by contact with packets of lens zonules. (Courtesy of Jonathan Herschler, M.D.)

204

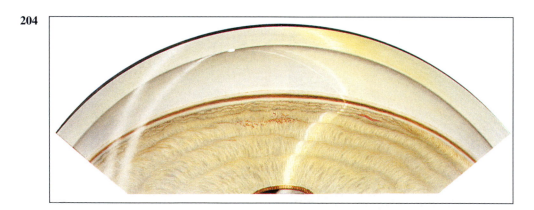

204 Patient with the pigment dispersion syndrome. The angle demonstrates a dense band of black pigment in the posterior trabecular meshwork.

After dilation pigmentation may be seen where the zonules attach to the posterior lens capsule. Pigment in this area is called a Scheie's stripe. Scheie's stripe can occasionally be seen with the slit lamp (**206**) but is best seen by gonioscopic examination (**207**).

205

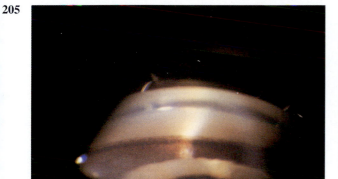

205 Marked posterior bowing in a patient with the pigment dispersion syndrome. Although a concave iris may be seen in the syndrome, this dramatic degree of concavity is unusual.

206

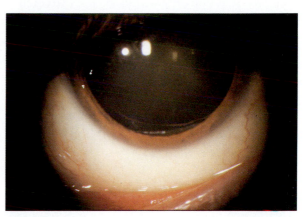

206 Scheie's stripe – a band of pigment at the junction of zonules and posterior lens capsule in the pigment dispersion syndrome seen at the inferior border of the pupil. The stripe is usually seen only gonioscopically.

207

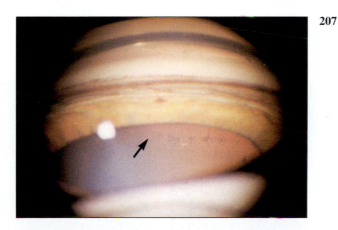

207 Scheie's stripe in the pigment dispersion syndrome. Pigment accumulates at the junction of the zonules and the posterior lens capsule (arrow). The trabecular meshwork is moderately pigmented.

Pseudoexfoliation (exfoliation syndrome, glaucoma capsulare) In pseudoexfoliation there is a deposition of basement membrane-like material throughout the anterior segment of the eye. Similar material has been identified at many other sites throughout the bodies of patients with pseudoexfoliation, but this material appears to cause dysfunction only within the eye (Streeten *et al.*, 1992). Eyes with pseudoexfoliation show an increased incidence of open-angle glaucoma and, occasionally, angle-closure glaucoma. This process can occur in one or both eyes and is a major cause of unilateral glaucoma. It occurs primarily among the elderly and is most prevalent among those of Scandinavian heritage.

On examination a granular or flaky deposit is observed on the anterior lens capsule, often with a clear zone where the iris has rubbed some of the deposited material off the lens (**208**). The edges of this material can curl at the pupillary border or

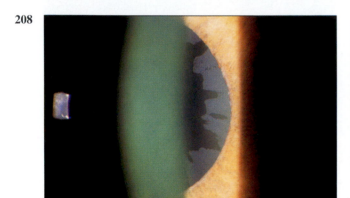

208 Slit-lamp photograph of pseudoexfoliative material on the anterior lens capsule. This material has a ground glass-like appearance and has areas that have been rubbed away by the motion of the iris against the lens capsule.

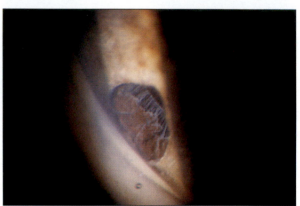

209 Gonioscopic view of pseudoexfoliative material on zonules. This view is through a peripheral iridectomy after a trabeculectomy. Note the frosted appearance of the zonules.

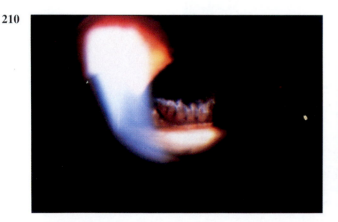

210 Gonioscopic photograph of pseudoexfoliative material on the ciliary body of an aphakic patient. (Courtesy of Richard K. Parrish II, MD, Bascom Palmer Eye Institute.)

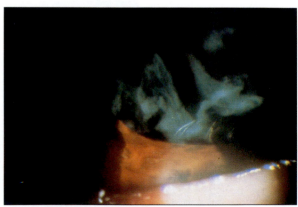

211 Pseudoexfoliation on the anterior vitreous face of an aphakic patient. (Courtesy of Paul F. Palmberg, MD, Ph.D, Bascom Palmer Eye Institute.)

can be seen there as dandruff-like debris. With transillumination patchy iris defects are often apparent at the pupillary border. Pigment may collect on the iris or corneal endothelium. The zonules are frosted with pseudoexfoliative material (**209**). The zonules are fragile, making zonular dehiscence a risk in extracapsular cataract extraction (Skuta *et al.*, 1987). In aphakic eyes pseudoexfoliative material may be seen on the ciliary processes (**210**) or on the face of the vitreous body (**211**).

Marked pigmentation of the angle is found on gonioscopic examination. The pigment typically has a more granular, brown character than the dense black pigment that is seen in the pigment dispersion syndrome (**212** and **213**).

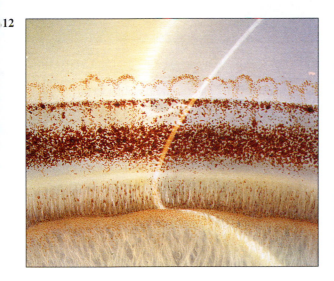

212 The angle in pseudoexfoliation. Note the clumped brown pigment over the pigmented trabecular meshwork. There is also a line of pigment along Schwalbe's line and another, wavy line of pigment anterior to this line.

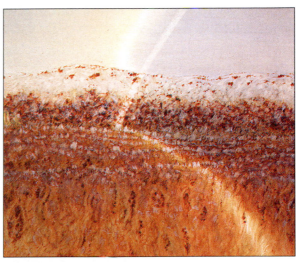

213 Pseudoexfoliation with a dense pigmentation of the angle that obscures most angle structures. The corneal wedge identifies Schwalbe's line.

Oculodermal melanocytosis In oculodermal melanocytosis there is abnormal pigmentation of the periorbital skin and globe. The involvement of the skin takes the form of a deep dermal pigmentation in the ophthalmic and maxillary distributions of the trigeminal nerve. If only the eye is affected the condition is termed melanosis oculi (**214**). Ocular pigmentation most commonly affects the episclera but may also involve the iris, fundus, conjunctiva, and trabecular meshwork (**215**). The disorder is more common in women than in men. It is seen most often in Orientals and other darkly pigmented individuals. Glaucoma has been reported in 10% of a large sample of patients with the condition (Teekhasaenee *et al.*, 1990).

Inspection of the angle of patients with glaucoma in oculodermal melanocytosis shows the trabecular meshwork to be covered by pigment or to be obscured by many pigmented iris processes (**216** and **217**). The ciliary body band is generally dark. The mechanism of glaucoma development is thought to be melanocytic infiltration of the trabecular meshwork and the dispersion of pigment. Evidence for the pigment dispersion mechanism is the finding of endothelial deposits of pigmentation with a Krukenberg spindle-like distribution (Teekhasaenee *et al.*, 1990).

214

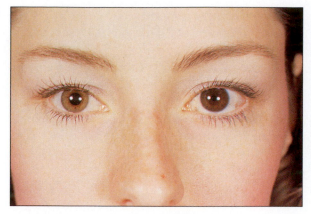

214 Heterochromia from melanosis oculi.

21

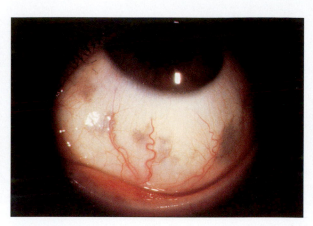

215 Deep slate-gray pigmentation of the episclera in a patient with melanosis oculi. There is also a dense pigmentation of the iris. (Same patient as **214**.)

216

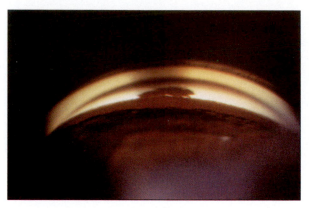

216 Gonioscopic view of the eye of a patient with melanosis oculi. There are abundant iris processes and marked pigmentation within the angle. (Courtesy of Robert Ritch, MD, New York Eye and Ear Infirmary.)

21

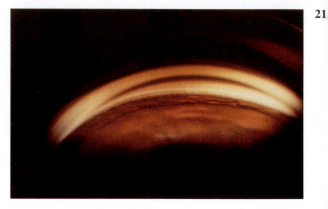

217 Normal fellow eye of patient shown in **216**. (Courtesy of Robert Ritch, MD, New York Eye and Ear Infirmary.)

Other causes of increased angle pigmentation
There may be a release of pigment after surgery. This can occur after incisional surgery (**218**) or after laser surgery. Peripheral laser iridotomy is a common cause of increased angle pigmentation, particularly of the inferior angle. Some patients with severe iridocyclitis may show a marked release of pigment into the anterior chamber (**219**). With angle closure there can be pigmentation of the angle from chronic iris contact. Melanomalytic glaucoma results from the release of pigment by a large melanoma, usually of the choroid. This is a very uncommon cause of increased angle pigmentation.

218 Gonioscopic view of temporal angle after cyclodialysis. Patients often have scattered pigmentation throughout the angle following surgery. The pigmentation is usually densest inferiorly.

218

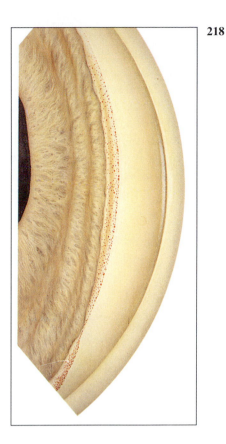

219

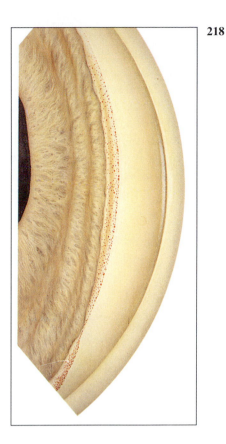

219 Dense trabecular pigmentation of the superior angle in a patient following herpes zoster ophthalmicus.

Blood

Blood may be observed in the anterior chamber secondary to a range of etiologies, such as trauma, surgery, and neovascularization. Blood settles into the inferior angle under the influence of gravity. Small amounts of blood can be seen onlyby gonioscopy (**220** and **221**). Small hyphemas do not usually result in an increase in intraocular pressure. Large hyphemas are more likely to cause problems with intraocular pressure as the trabecular meshwork fills with blood. Very large hyphemas that extend into the posterior chamber can occlude the pupil and cause elevated pressure secondary to pupillary block. In some patients with recurring hyphemas – especially following surgery – gonioscopy can be used to locate bleeding vessels and to treat them with a laser. Small balls of pigment may be seen in the angle long after a hyphema has resolved (*see* **247**).

220

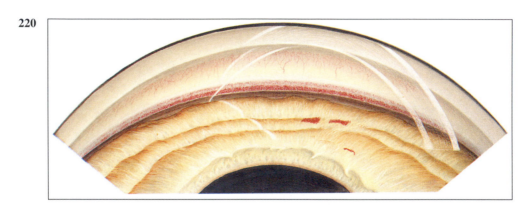

220 Gonioscopic view of inferior angle in a 16-year-old boy who was struck in the eye. There is blood lying on the trabecular meshwork.

221

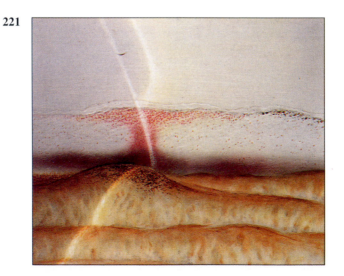

221 A higher-magnification gonioscopic view of the inferior angle of the eye of a 17-year-old boy shortly after he was struck in the eye. There is a small amount of blood anterior to the trabecular meshwork and also in Schlemm's canal.

Ghost-cell glaucoma is an unusual disorder that is seen in patients with vitreous hemorrhage. Red blood cells denature within the vitreous body and take on a spherical form, in contrast to the normal biconcave shape (**222**). The cells are inflexible and pass through the trabecular meshwork with difficulty (Campbell *et al.*, 1976). Such cells are more likely to raise intraocular pressure than red blood cells. Ghost erythrocytes may be identified by their characteristic khaki color on slit-lamp (**223**) and gonioscopic examination. Glaucoma is most likely to develop in aphakic eyes or in eyes with zonular breaks through which the ghost cells can gain access to the anterior chamber.

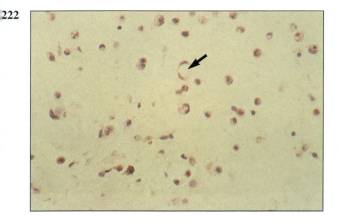

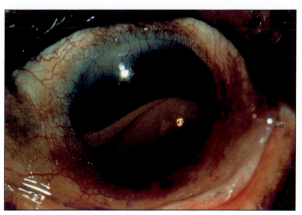

222 Ghost erythrocytes from the vitreous body of a patient with chronic intraocular hemorrhage. The cells are spherical with marginated denatured hemoglobin (arrow).

223 Ghost cells in the anterior chamber of an aphakic patient. Note the candy stripe of bright red cells within the degenerated khaki-colored cells. (Courtesy of David G. Campbell. Previously published in: M. Bruce Shields, MD, *Textbook of Glaucoma,* Williams and Wilkins, Baltimore, 1992. Used with permission.)

Inflammation

In the inflamed eye one can see precipitates on the internal cornea and on the trabecular meshwork. Sometimes the precipitates are revealed only by gonioscopic examination (**224**). Small hypopyons may be visible in the inferior angle with gonioscopy. Peripheral anterior synechiae are frequently observed after chronic inflammation as large precipitates consolidate (**225** and **226**) and cause the iris to become adherent to the trabecular meshwork. Closure of the angle by synechiae is discussed in Chapter 8.

Fuchs' heterochromic iridocyclitis is a form of inflammatory glaucoma with a unique constellation of findings. Examination reveals: frequent heterochromia (**227** and **228**), mild inflammation

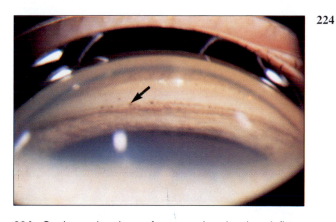

224 Gonioscopic view of an angle showing inflammatory precipitates (arrow) on the trabecular meshwork. (Published courtesy of E. Michael Van Buskirk, MD, *Clinical Atlas of Glaucoma.* W. B. Saunders, Philadelphia, 1986.)

of the anterior chamber, diffuse fine stellate keratic precipitates (**229** and **230**), cataract (**231**), and neovascularization of the iris (**232**) and angle (**233**). These fine angle vessels do not often lead to the development of synechiae. The vessels are very fragile and can bleed on paracentesis of the anterior chamber (Amsler and Verrey, 1946) and even on gonioscopy (Begg, 1969). The most consistent feature of Fuchs' heterochromic iridocyclitis is a flat, featureless iris (**228** and **234**) (Kimura *et al.*, 1955).

Glaucomatocyclitic crisis is an uncommon unilateral mild inflammation accompanied by strikingly elevated intraocular pressures of 40–60

225
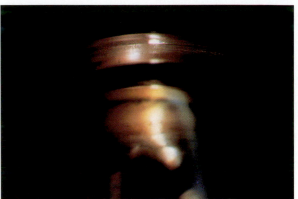

225 Slit-lamp photograph showing a large sarcoid granuloma in the inferior angle. This inflammatory mass can consolidate and pull the iris over the trabecular meshwork.

226 Gonioscopic view of a sarcoid granuloma of the inferior angle. Same patient as in **225**.

227
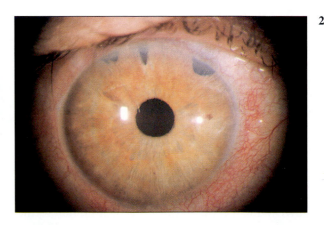

228

227 Normal right eye of a patient who has Fuchs' heterochromic iridocyclitis in the left eye.

228 Left eye of the patient in **227**. This eye has Fuchs' heterochromic iridocyclitis. Note the surgical iridectomies from filtration surgery and also the hypochromia of this iris when compared with the right eye. The iris is flat and featureless and lacks the normal crypts seen in the other eye.

mm Hg. There are often a few small, colorless keratic precipitates over the inferior corneal endothelium. There may be slight pupillary dilation and iris hypochromia is occasionally observed on the affected side. The high pressure can cause corneal edema. The angle is open and has normal pigmentation. Synechiae do not develop (Posner and Schlossman, 1948). The sudden, strikingly high intraocular pressure rises can lead to a mistaken diagnosis of acute angle closure unless gonioscopy is performed.

A rare syndrome of precipitates on the trabecular meshwork was described by Chandler and Grant in 1965. This presents like primary open-

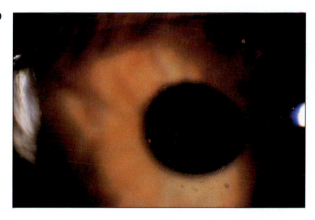

229 Same patient as **227** and **228**. A closer view of the left eye demonstrates diffuse, small, keratic precipitates over the entire corneal endothelium.

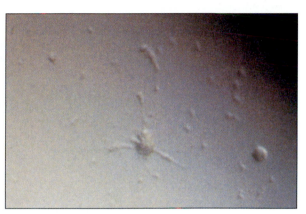

230 A high-magnification view of a keratic precipitate in Fuchs' heterochromic iridocyclitis. Note that the precipitate is clear and has dendritic projections. (W. L. M. Alward, MD, Uveitic Glaucoma. In: Tasman, W., and Jaeger, E. A., eds, *Clinical Ophthalmology.* Courtesy of J.B. Lippincott, Philadelphia, 1989.)

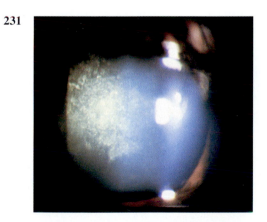

231 Posterior subcapsular cataract in Fuchs' heterochromic iridocyclitis. (Bascom Palmer Eye Institute.)

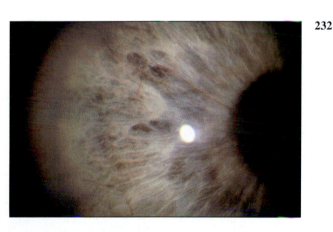

232 Diffuse neovascularization of the iris in Fuchs' heterochromic iridocyclitis.

angle glaucoma but demonstrates a paradoxical increase in intraocular pressure with cholinergic agents. On examination fine inflammatory precipitates are seen on the trabecular meshwork (as in **224**). The eye is otherwise generally quiet. The pressure usually responds to corticosteroids and aqueous suppressants, but recurrences are the rule and patients frequently require indefinite therapy. Some cases develop full-blown inflammation of the anterior chamber, while others never experience inflammation beyond the trabecular meshwork. Synechiae are a common development.

233

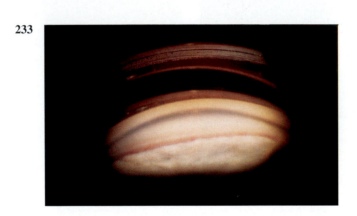

233 Neovascularization of the angle in Fuchs' heterochromic iridocyclitis. These vessels are extremely fragile and bleed with minor trauma. Unlike other forms of neovascularization, the tendency to form synechiae is minimal.

234

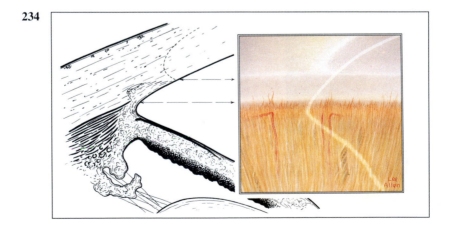

234 Gonioscopic view showing flat, featureless iris with neovascularization in Fuchs' heterochromic iridocyclitis.

Lens material

When the lens is ruptured the fragments may cause obstruction of the aqueous outflow. In lens-particle glaucoma a fine glistening can be seen in the angle due to the presence of lens fragments (235 and 236). Fragments of lens are identified on tapping the anterior chamber.

Phacolytic glaucoma is seen in eyes with mature or hypermature cataracts (237). The affected lenses leak denatured protein through an intact capsule into the anterior chamber. Macrophages engulf the material and are seen floating in the anterior chamber amid a heavy

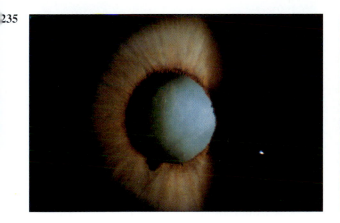

235 Patient with recent trauma demonstrating a tear of the sphincter. The patient had a marked elevation of his intraocular pressure.

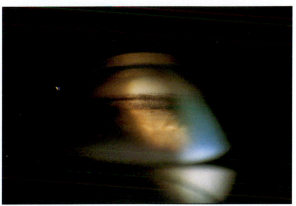

236 Gonioscopic view of the eye shown in **235**. The patient had glistening material on the surface of the trabecular meshwork. An anterior chamber tap demonstrated lens particles. Note that the angle is probably recessed.

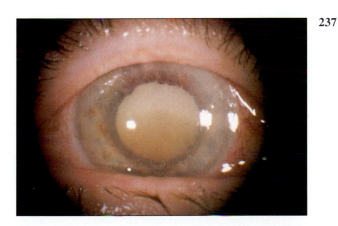

237 A hypermature cataract with a liquefied cortex and a brunescent nucleus that has sunk to the inferior portion of the lens.

238

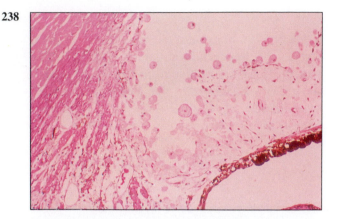

238 Phacolytic glaucoma in an eye with traumatic angle recession and a hypermature lens. Lens protein-filled macrophages are identified in the recessed angle. (Courtesy of Robert Folberg, MD, University of Iowa.)

239

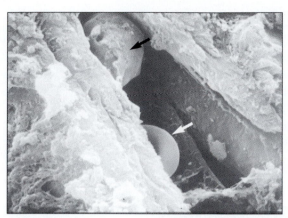

239 Scanning electron micrograph of intratrabecular space from an eye with phacolytic glaucoma. A red blood cell (white arrow) and a macrophage (black arrow) are seen between the trabecular pillars. Note the ruffled surface of the macrophage. (Courtesy of Robert Folberg, MD, University of Iowa.)

flare. White material observed on the anterior lens capsule probably represents collections of macrophages. The trabecular meshwork becomes obstructed by macrophages (**238** and **239**) and protein (Epstein *et al.*, 1978). Pressure elevation is often abrupt and can reach very high levels. The eye is usually injected and the cornea is frequently edematous.

Foreign bodies

Foreign bodies can be found lodged in the anterior chamber angle after trauma (**240** and **241**). They are usually located in the inferior angle and may be found on routine examination. Most are inert and damage the eye only if they traumatize the corneal endothelium. If a patient presents with focal corneal edema, gonioscopy may reveal that a foreign body has lodged in the angle. When such bodies are removed the edema usually clears (McDonald and Ashodian, 1959). Some metallic

240

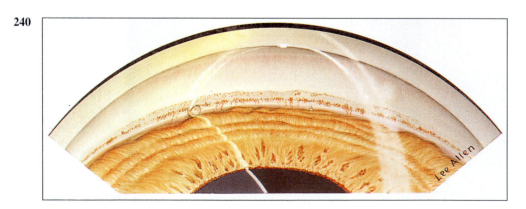

240 Sand in the inferior angle after a land-mine explosion.

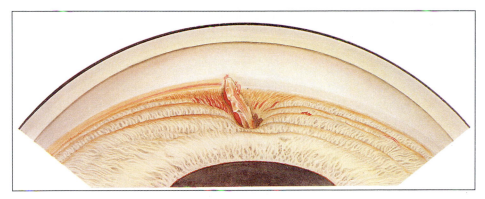

241 Glass in the inferior angle after trauma. The patient had broken his glasses while working in a sawmill. A fragment of glass was removed earlier. The patient presented with discomfort and injection. The chip of glass is wedged between the trabecular meshwork and the iris, distorting both structures. There is a small tear in the iris and clotted blood under the fragment. Some blood is present in Schlemm's canal.

and vegetable foreign materials are poorly tolerated. Siderosis is a late effect of a retained foreign body composed of iron or steel. The iron oxidizes and ions are dispersed through the eye, resulting in toxicity to the trabecular meshwork, lens, cornea, and retina. The trabecular meshwork may take on a rusty hue (**242**) and the eye may develop late glaucoma. The most striking slit-lamp finding is a rust-colored anterior cataract (**243**). The most serious effects of siderosis arise from toxicity to the retina.

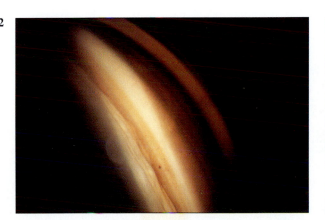

242 The angle of a 28-year-old man who was struck in the eye by a metal clip from a concrete form. He sustained an intraocular iron foreign body. Note the rusty discoloration of the trabecular meshwork from siderosis.

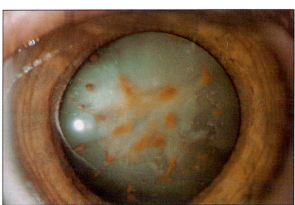

243 Cataract from siderosis in an eye with a retained iron foreign body.

Traumatic Angle Changes

Iridodialysis

Iridodialyses, or tears in the iris (**244–246**), occur as the result of blunt trauma. Bleeding from the tears can result in hyphemas. By themselves iridodialyses generally cause no problems. Occasionally there will be some flattening of the pupil in the quadrant of the tear. Some patients may notice extra images through the iris defect.

An iridodialysis mostly serves as an indicator that the eye has previously sustained a substantial impact and should alert one to the possibility of angle recession or retinal damage. Some iridodialyses occur so far towards the periphery that they can be appreciated only by gonioscopy.

 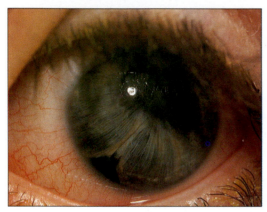

244 Inferior iridodialysis following trauma.

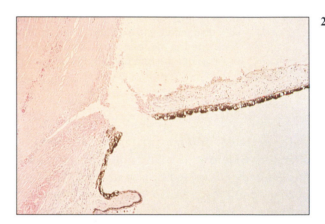

245 Histopathologic view of iridodialysis showing a tear through the peripheral iris. The normal iris is thinnest at its insertion into the ciliary body. (Courtesy of Robert Folberg, M.D., University of Iowa.)

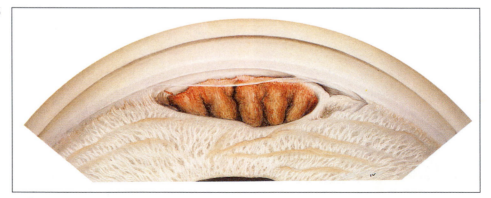

246 Gonioscopic view of traumatic iridodialysis in the inferior angle found on routine examination. The patient remembered having sustained blunt trauma to the eye several years previously. Ciliary processes can be seen through the iris defect.

Angle recession

A recessed angle occurs as a result of severe blunt trauma in which there is a tear in the face of the ciliary body, usually between the longitudinal and circular muscles. The tear can occur over a limited area or may involve the entire angle. Angle recession is important because of the accompanying increased risk of glaucoma. Glaucoma occurs in about 9% of patients with recessed angles and may develop months or years after the injury (Kaufman and Tolpin, 1974). Most patients with significant hyphemas will be found to have angle recession after the hemorrhage clears (Tonjum, 1966).

Gonioscopic examination shows a wide ciliary body band and a deep anterior chamber (**247** and **248**). It is useful to compare eyes to determine if one eye has an abnormally wide ciliary body band. The ciliary face may appear lighter in the recessed area because there is little ciliary tissue overlying the sclera (**247** and **249**). The presence of torn tissue may give the ciliary face a cobweb appearance. Iris processes will be broken and the scleral spur may appear whiter than normal because the uveal meshwork has been torn from the surface.

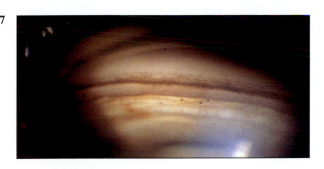

247 Angle of a 45-year-old man who was hit with a BB as a child. He later developed unilateral glaucoma from angle recession. Note the very deep anterior chamber and the large amount of ciliary body face visible below the scleral spur. The ciliary body band is a light color because it consists of only a thin layer of tissue over sclera. The tiny black balls on the iris are residuals from old hemorrhage.

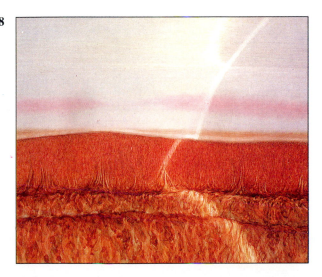

248 Angle recession in an 11-year-old who was struck in the eye. Note the step-off below the scleral spur and the deep ciliary body face. There is blood in Schlemm's canal.

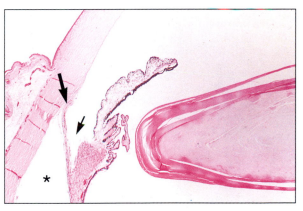

249 Histopathology of angle recession showing a tear in the anterior face of the ciliary body between the longitudinal and circular fibers (small arrow). The ciliary body is still attached to the scleral spur (large arrow). The space between sclera and the ciliary body (*) is an artifact. (Courtesy of Robert Folberg, MD, University of Iowa.)

Cyclodialysis cleft

A cyclodialysis cleft is the dis-insertion of the ciliary body from the scleral spur. This permits free access of aqueous into the suprachoroidal space and usually results in decreased intraocular pressure. Cyclodialysis clefts can occur as a result of trauma or can be created surgically. Surgical cyclodialysis is rarely performed now because of problems with hemorrhage and hypotony and the failure to provide long-term control.

A cyclodialysis cleft appears as a very deep angle with a cleft through which the white color of the sclera is visible (**250** and **252**). As in angle recession, there will be rupture of any iris processes in the area of the cleft and the scleral spur may appear to be whiter than in other areas.

A cyclodialysis cleft is a detachment of the ciliary body from the scleral spur (**251**), while a recessed angle is a tear into the face of the ciliary body. A comparison of the histopathology shown in **249** and **251** illustrates this difference clearly.

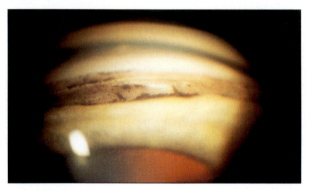

250 Gonioscopic view of the angle of a patient following trauma. A cyclodialysis cleft is seen as a white band below the trabecular meshwork. The chamber angle is very deep. This patient suffered from hypotony, which resolved following argon-laser treatment to the area around the cleft.

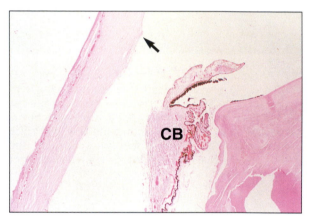

251 Histopathologic section of a cyclodialysis cleft showing the dis-insertion of the ciliary body (**CB**) from the scleral spur (arrow). (Courtesy of Robert Folberg, MD, University of Iowa.)

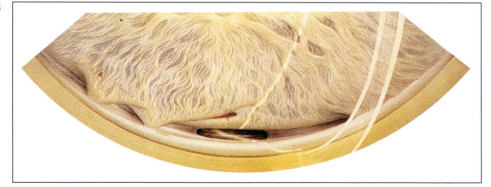

252 Aphakic glaucoma status after surgical cyclodialysis showing an open cleft with surrounding synechiae.

Angle recession is associated with a normal or elevated intraocular pressure, whereas a cyclodialysis cleft is associated with a normal or decreased intraocular pressure.

Cyclodialysis clefts may close spontaneously or they can be closed surgically. In both cases there may be a dramatic elevation of intraocular pressure.

Tumors

Tumors of the posterior segment, iris, and ciliary body can elevate intraocular pressure by closing the angle, as discussed in Chapter 8. Open-angle mechanisms by which tumors can elevate pressure include tumor seeding into the angle, a ring melanoma, or shedding of pigment from a large choroidal melanoma (melanomalytic glaucoma) (Yanoff, 1970).

Glaucoma occurs more frequently with tumors of the anterior segment, particularly malignant melanoma. Uveal malignant melanomas of the anterior segment lead to the development of glaucoma in over 41% of cases – compared to 14% of posterior melanomas (Yanoff, 1970).

Eyes with melanomas of the anterior segment associated with glaucoma have a poorer prognosis than eyes in which glaucoma has not developed (Shields and Klintworth, 1980). Other tumors of the anterior segment can cause glaucoma, but less commonly than melanoma.

A gonioscopic examination is critical in evaluating the extent of tumor involvement in eyes with malignancies of the anterior segment. The examination may reveal a direct invasion of the angle (253 and 254). Even if this is not demonstrated, diffuse invasion of the angle cannot be ruled out (255–257).

253

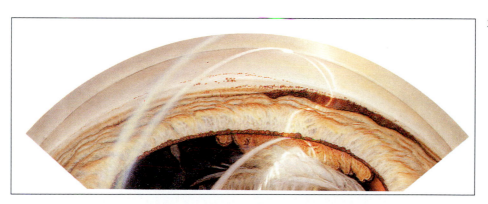

253 Gonioscopic view of malignant melanoma of the ciliary body invading through the iris into the angle.

254

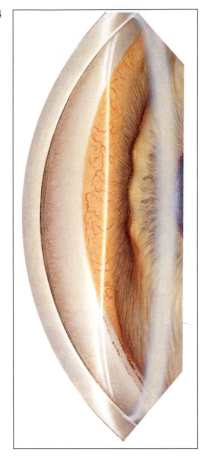

254 Large malignant melanoma of the ciliary body extending into the anterior segment and covering the nasal angle.

255

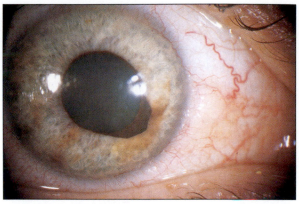

255 Slit-lamp photograph of inferonasal mass of the iris with ectropion uvea. This patient suffered from elevated intraocular pressure and very poor vision due to glaucoma.

256

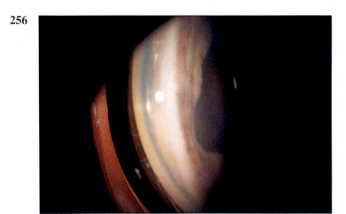

256 On gonioscopy the mass seen in **255** does not appear to extend into the chamber angle.

257

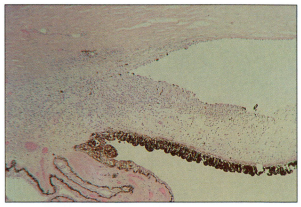

257 On histopathology, the mass seen in **255** and **256** is found to be a malignant melanoma affecting the iris root, trabecular meshwork and ciliary body through 360°.

Blood in Schlemm's Canal

The presence of blood in Schlemm's canal (**258**) may be caused by an abnormal flow relationship between the anterior chamber and the episcleral venous channels. The normal episcleral venous pressure is 8–10 mm Hg and the normal intra-ocular pressure is 10–21 mm Hg. The higher intraocular pressure normally causes aqueous flow to be directed towards the venous system. If the episcleral venous pressure is higher than the intraocular pressure, blood flows into Schlemm's canal. This can occur with intraorbital or intracranial vascular abnormalities such as carotid–cavernous fistulas, dural-sinus fistulas, Sturge–Weber syndrome, etc. In these conditions conjunctival and episcleral vessels are usually dilated and tortuous (**259**). If the eye is hypo-tonous blood will also reflux into Schlemm's canal. If a Goldmann lens is pressed too tightly against the globe, episcleral venous outflow will be impeded and blood will appear in the canal. Blood can also be seen in Schlemm's canal in some normal eyes.

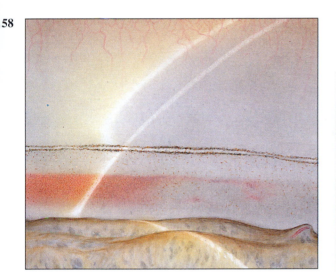

258 Gonioscopic view of an angle showing blood in Schlemm's canal. There is, incidentally, a prominent Schwalbe's line.

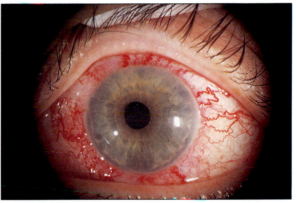

259 Engorged, tortuous blood vessels in a patient with elevated episcleral venous pressure due to a low-flow dural-sinus fistula.

Post-Surgical Changes

Many changes occur in the angle following surgery to the anterior segment. After surgery for glaucoma gonioscopy is a valuable tool for examining the surgical site. A patent internal sclerostomy should be visible after a trabeculec-tomy or a full-thickness filter (**260**). In some cases the iris or ciliary body may become incar-cerated (**260**). In iridencleisis some iris tissue is intentionally pulled into the edges of the wound (**261**). Setons are usually visible with the slit lamp, but they may be located so far into the angle that gonioscopy is necessary to evaluate the location and patency of the tube (**262**).

After cataract extraction the anterior chamber

260

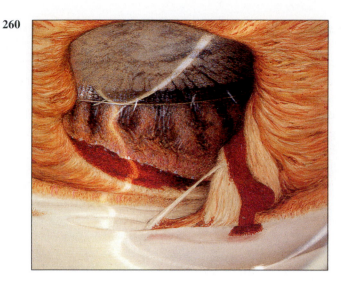

260 Angle after trabeculectomy with incarceration of uveal material into the filtering sclerostomy.

261

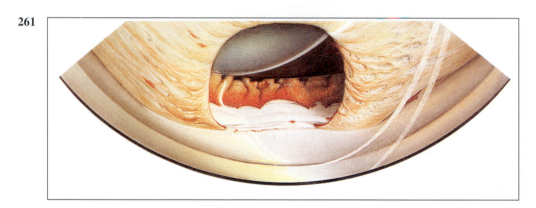

261 Gonioscopic view of iridencleisis showing an opened fistula into which leaves of iris are tucked.

262

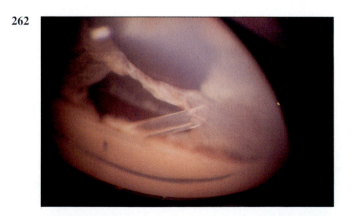

262 Gonioscopic view of tube from Baerveldt seton within the anterior chamber.

is generally quite deep because of the loss of lens thickness (**263**). The cataract wound can be visualized internally (**264**). Many ocular structures may become incarcerated in the cataract wound, for example zonules (**264**), iris (**265**), or vitreous body (**266**). One may see evidence of traumatic changes resulting from surgery, such as a scroll of detached Descemet's membrane (**267**). In an eye with an anterior chamber intraocular lens gonioscopy can be helpful in evaluating the placement of the haptics (**268** and **269**).

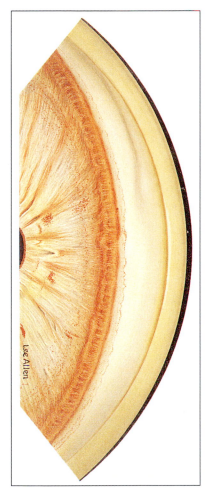

263 Nasal angle of aphakic eye showing a deep anterior chamber, which is common after the removal of a lens. There is deep pigmentation in the trabecular meshwork. The cataract wound can be seen in the top half of the cornea.

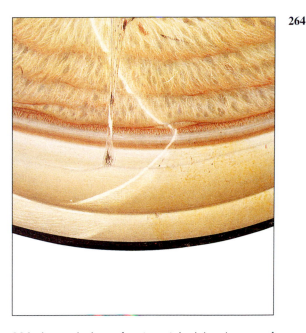

264 Internal view of cataract incision in eye of aphakic patient. A small strand of zonular fibers adheres to the wound.

265

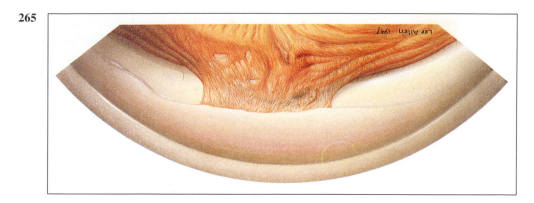

265 A large band of iris incarcerated in a cataract wound. The painting is positioned to show the superior angle viewed through an indirect lens. The artist's name therefore appears upside down.

266

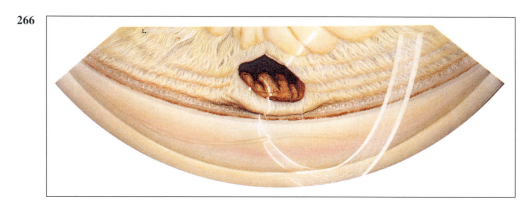

266 Gonioscopic view after intracapsular cataract extraction showing a sheet of vitreous that passes through the iridectomy and into the wound.

267

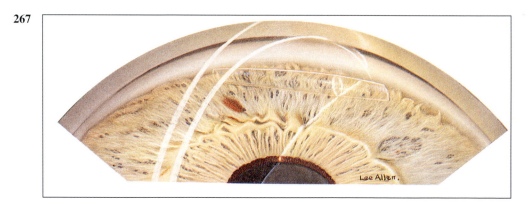

267 Inferior scroll of Descemet's membrane after surgery.

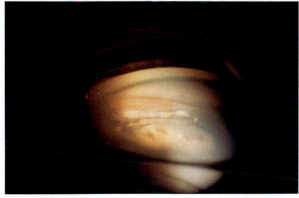

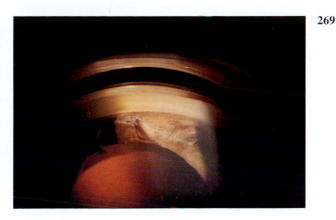

268 Haptics of an anterior chamber lens in the anterior chamber angle.

269 Haptics of an anterior chamber lens in the chamber angle. Note that the haptic to the left is embedded in the anterior surface of the iris.

Miscellaneous Conditions

Iris-retraction syndrome

The rare iris-retraction syndrome occurs when a rhegmatogenous retinal detachment occurs in an eye with a secluded pupil (Campbell, 1984). Patients with secluded pupils develop iris bombé as aqueous humor trapped in the posterior chamber pushes the iris forward. When there is a rhegmatogenous retinal detachment there is some flow of aqueous through the break. If patients with secluded pupils and rhegmatogenous retinal detachments are placed on aqueous suppressants they may make so little aqueous humor that it is all able to flow through the retinal break, causing the iris to be pulled back – often dramatically (**270** and **271**) If aqueous suppressants are discontinued the eye may develop iris bombé again (Campbell, 1984).

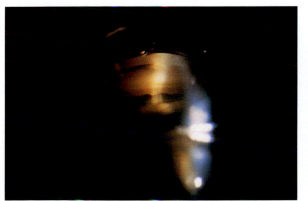

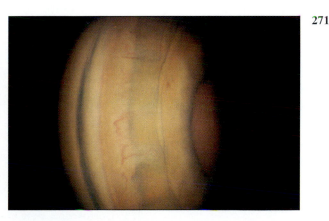

270 Patient with a rhegmatogenous retinal detachment and secluded pupil. When treated with acetazolamide the patient developed a marked back-bowing of the iris, typical of the iris-retraction syndrome. The markedly concave shape of the iris should be noted.

271 Iris-retraction syndrome. Eye of the same patient as in **270**, seen here with diffuse illumination and higher magnification. Note that the iris is pulled very far posteriorly and iris vessels are exposed and stretched.

Corneal disease

Some corneal diseases can be examined gonioscopically. External tumors can be seen through the cornea (**272**) and one can evaluate for internal spread. The vasculature of interstitial keratitis can be visualized (**273**).

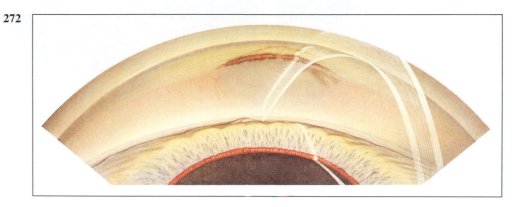

272 A patient with melanoma at the limbus visible by gonioscopy. The patient had had a small pigmented spot at the limbus since birth. Over the preceding nine months the spot had enlarged and grown on to her cornea. After gonioscopic examination the tumor was locally excised and found to be a malignant melanoma.

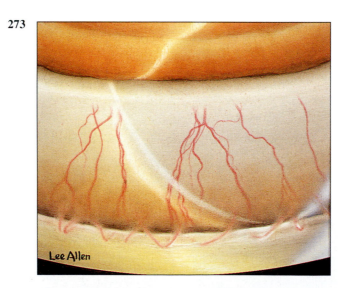

273 Gonioscopic view of eye of patient with interstitial keratitis showing blood vessels in the cornea that are visible only to the level of the trabecular meshwork.

10 Gonioscopic Laser Surgery

Both laser and incisional surgery are performed with the aid of gonioscopic visualization of the angle. Incisional surgery includes goniotomy, goniosynechialysis, internally created filtration procedures, and internal revisions of filtration fistulas. Such procedures are performed by only a small proportion of ophthalmologists and fall outside the scope of this atlas. Gonioscopic lenses are used more often for laser surgery than for incisional surgery. The most common gonioscopic laser procedures are trabeculoplasty, iridoplasty, and cyclophotocoagulation of the ciliary body. These three procedures will be discussed in some detail. More recently, *ab interno* laser fistulas and laser lysis of synechiae have been described. These procedures have not reached general use and are not discussed.

Laser Trabeculoplasty

Argon-laser trabeculoplasty is the most frequently performed procedure for glaucoma. It successfully lowers intraocular pressure in about 80% of patients with primary open-angle glaucoma (Thomas *et al.,* 1982). The mean drop in pressure is about 10 mm Hg and is proportional to that before treatment (Thomas *et al.,* 1982; Wise and Witter, 1979). Laser trabeculoplasty is efficacious in treating primary open-angle glaucoma and some secondary open-angle glaucomas, such as those associated with pseudoexfoliation and the pigment dispersion syndrome. It is less successful in patients with infantile glaucoma, angle recession, inflammatory glaucoma, and aphakia and in young patients (Thomas *et al.,* 1982; Wise and Witter, 1979).

A Goldmann three-mirror lens is usually used for trabeculoplasty. The lens should have an anti-reflective coating to allow maximum delivery of the laser energy to the angle. Some ophthalmologists prefer to use the Ritch lens, which has magnifying 'buttons' to focus the laser energy on to a smaller area. The Ritch lens also has mirrors that are designed specifically for the superior and inferior angles (Ritch, 1985).

An understanding of the anatomy of the angle is a critical requirement for performing argon-laser trabeculoplasty. The burns are applied at the junction of the pigmented and non-pigmented trabecular meshwork (**274**). Delivery of laser energy too far posteriorly results in increased inflammation and an increased number of peripheral anterior synechiae (Rouhiainen *et al.,* 1988) (*see* **190** and **191**). Laser energy delivered too far anteriorly may result in overgrowth of the trabecular meshwork by corneal endothelium (Rodrigues *et al.,* 1982). The techniques described in Chapter 4 can be used to help define the anatomy. If the angle is confusing one should look inferiorly at the deepest and most pigmented portion of the angle to become oriented to the patient's anatomy. The corneal wedge can be invaluable in determining the location of Schwalbe's line. In patients on miotics with steep approaches to the angle dilation can be used to improve the visibility of the angle. In patients with a poor view of the angle secondary to pupillary block one may need to perform a peripheral iridotomy with a laser. In eyes with plateau iris configuration and in other cases where the angle is crowded it may be helpful to perform iridoplasty before carrying out trabeculoplasty.

It can be difficult to maintain one's bearings while performing laser trabeculoplasty because of the mirrored view of the angle. If a long series of laser spots is delivered and the lens is then rotated for a second series of spots, it is easy to become lost unless there are visible angle landmarks such as iris processes, nevi, or distinct laser burns. I prefer to hold the Goldmann lens with three fingers (**55**) and rotate the lens slightly after every few applications, keeping the area undergoing treatment in the center of the mirror.

A 50-μm spot of argon blue–green or green light is normally used. The duration of delivery is 0.1 s. The power required varies from 200 to 1200 mW and is adjusted until an adequate uptake of energy is noted. In an angle with average pigmentation I generally start with approximately 700 mW. In a darkly pigmented angle, as found in cases of pseudoexfoliation and pigmentary glaucoma, I begin with approximately 300 mW. In extremely lightly pigmented angles no visible uptake of laser energy may be apparent despite a power level of 1200 mW. An adequate response to treatment is signified by blanching or the formation of small bubbles in the trabecular meshwork (**274**). If a crater, a large bubble, or a shower of bubbles forms the intensity is too high. The use of power levels greater than 1000–1200 mW is not recommended. If there is no visible response at 1200 mW, I complete the treatment at this level. A therapeutic effect may result even if no visible angle changes occur.

274

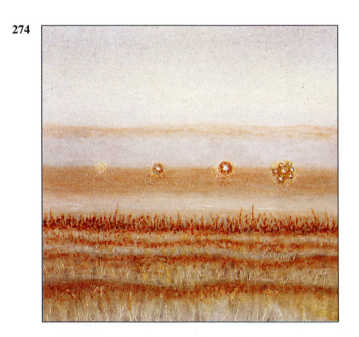

274 Burns induced by argon-laser trabeculoplasty. The burns are placed at the junction of the pigmented and non-pigmented portions of the trabecular meshwork. The end-point is a blanching of the meshwork (left) or a small bubble (second from left). A large bubble (second from right) or a shower of bubbles (right) indicates that excessive laser energy is being applied.

It is important to have the burn strike the trabecular meshwork perpendicularly. When properly aligned, a crisp round spot will be formed by the aiming beam. This is easiest to judge if the aiming beam is kept fairly dim. If the spot is distorted or oblong the Goldmann lens is probably being held at an unusual angle. It is often helpful to look around the slit-lamp oculars and adjust the lens so that the front surface is parallel to the plane of the patient's face. This should help to give a distinct, round spot. In the case of patients with steep approaches to the trabecular meshwork who are looking into the mirror in order to allow the physician to treat the meshwork there will be some distortion of the beam because of the angle of approach. A flatter approach, parallel to the iris, is preferred. Some authors suggest that the patient should be asked to look slightly away from the mirror so that a flat approach into the meshwork can be obtained (Palmberg, 1989). With most patients, however, satisfactory results are obtained if they look straight ahead through the entire procedure. Laser trabeculoplasty can be performed over 180° or 360°. Typically, 40–50 laser applications are applied over each 180°.

The most common complication from laser trabeculoplasty is postoperative elevation of the intraocular pressure. Apraclonidine has been shown to decrease the number and intensity of pressure spikes markedly after laser trabeculoplasty and is generally administered at the time of the procedure (Robin *et al.*, 1987). There should be postoperative monitoring for intraocular pressure spikes.

Retreatment of a previously treated angle has met with varying success. Although some authors have found retreatment to be safe and efficacious in selected patients (Jorizzo *et al.*, 1988), others have reported an unacceptable number of pressure spikes and a low success rate (Brown *et al.*, 1985). I have had few patients for whom I have found repeat trabeculoplasty indicated.

Laser Iridoplasty

Laser iridoplasty is used to pull the iris away from the angle. This is done in eyes with plateau iris configuration – when argon-laser trabeculoplasty is difficult due to a crowded angle – and, rarely, in eyes with acute angle closure in which laser iridotomy cannot be performed. Laser iridoplasty can be performed either through a Goldmann three-mirror lens or directly through the cornea without the use of a lens, aiming at the most peripheral iris (**275**). I prefer the latter technique. In either case iridoplasty is done with large, slowly applied spots of low power. This power is chosen to shrink, not perforate, the iris. Spots of 200–500 μm with durations of 0.2–0.5 s are used. The power is adjusted until visible shrinkage is noted; this usually requires power settings of 150–300 mW.

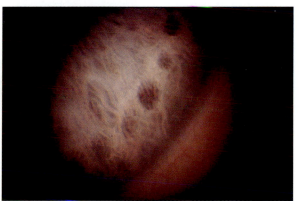

275

275 Scars from argon-laser iridoplasty. The energy was administered through the cornea without a gonioscopic lens in this patient with plateau iris syndrome.

Laser Cyclophotocoagulation

Many techniques for the destruction of the ciliary body have been described. Laser energy for cyclophotocoagulation can be delivered through an endoscope, trans-sclerally, or through a gonioscopic lens. Transpupillary photocoagulation in humans was first described by Merritt in 1976. Laser energy is delivered through a Goldmann three-mirror lens. Merritt described the use of indentation to bring the ciliary body processes into view to allow treatment. In most cases cyclophotocoagulation through the pupil requires an extremely large pupil, a sector iridectomy, or aniridia. Most patients with glaucoma have small pupils secondary to the use of cholinergic agents, which eliminates the possibility of transpupillary cyclophotocoagulation. Patients with aniridia would seem to be ideal candidates for this procedure. Unfortunately, most patients with congenital aniridia have developed corneal pannus by the time their glaucoma requires cyclophotocoagulation.

A spot size of 50–200 μm is used with a duration of 0.1–0.2 s and a power setting of 700–1000 mW. 90° to 180° of the ciliary body is treated. The power is increased until the ciliary processes demonstrate shrinkage and whitening (**276**). All visible processes in one or two quadrants are treated. Postoperatively, the eye is treated with corticosteroids and cycloplegics. Transpupillary cyclophotocoagulation tends to treat the anterior portion of the ciliary body. It is difficult to treat the posterior portion, where most of the aqueous humor is produced (Shields *et al.*, 1985b). In my experience it is uncommon to be able to treat enough of the ciliary body in this way to lower intraocular pressure permanently.

276

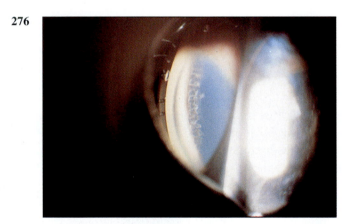

276 Gonioscopic view of the ciliary body of a patient with traumatic aniridia. Transpupillary cyclophotocoagulation was previously performed with the argon laser. Note the whitening of the treated ciliary processes. (Alward, W. L. M., in Weingeist, T. A. and Sneed, S.R. eds. *Laser Surgery in Ophthalmology: Practical Applications.* 1992. Published courtesy of Appleton and Lange, Norwalk.)

References

Allen, J. H., and Allen, L. (1950). Buried muscle cone implant: development of tunneled hemispheric type. *Arch. Ophthalmol.,* **43:** 879–890.

Allen, L. (1944). New contact lens for viewing angle of anterior chamber of eye. *Science,* **99:** 186.

Allen, L. (1964a). Ocular fundus photography: suggestions for achieving consistently good pictures and instructions for stereoscopic photography. *Am. J. Ophthalmol.,* **57:** 13–28.

Allen, L. (1964b). Stereoscopic fundus photography with the new instant positive print films. *Am. J. Ophthalmol.,* **57:** 539–543.

Allen, L., Braley, A. E., *et al.* (1954). An improved gonioscopic contact prism. *Arch. Ophthalmol.,* **51:** 451–455.

Allen, L., and Burian, H. M. (1961). The trabeculotome: an instrument for trabeculotomy ab externo. *Trans. Am. Acad. Ophthalmol. Otolaryngol.,* **65:** 200–201.

Allen, L., and Burian, H. M. (1962). Trabeculotomy ab externo. A new glaucoma operation: technique and results of experimental surgery. *Am. J. Ophthalmol.,* **53:** 19–26.

Allen, L., and Burian, H. M. (1965). The valve action of the trabecular meshwork. *Am. J. Ophthalmol.,* **59:** 382–389.

Allen, L., Burian, H. M., *et al.* (1955). The anterior border ring of Schwalbe and the pectinate ligament. *Arch. Ophthalmol.,* **53:** 799–806.

Allen, L., Ferguson, E. C., *et al.* (1960). A quasi-integrated buried muscle cone implant with good motility and advantages for prosthetic fitting. *Trans. Am. Acad. Ophthalmol. Otolaryngol.,* **64:** 272–286.

Allen, L., and O'Brien, C. S. (1945). Gonioscopy simplified by a contact prism. *Arch. Ophthalmol.,* **34:** 413–414.

American Academy of Ophthalmology (1989). Clinical Alert 2/4: Updated recommendations for ophthalmic practice in relation to the human immunodeficiency virus. *Ophthalmology,* **96:** 1–2.

Amsler, M., and Verrey, F. (1946). Heterochromia of Fuchs' and vascular fragility. *Ophthalmologica,* **111:** 178–181.

Anderson, D. R. (1981). The development of the trabecular meshwork and its abnormality in primary infantile glaucoma. *Trans. Am. Ophthalmol. Soc.,* **79:** 458–485.

Barkan, O. (1937). Recent advances in the surgery of chronic glaucoma. *Am. J. Ophthalmol.,* **20:** 1237–1245.

Barkan, O. (1938). Glaucoma: classification, causes, and surgical control. Results of microgonioscopic research. *Am. J. Ophthalmol.,* **21:** 1099–1117.

Barkan, O., Boyle, S. F., *et al.* (1936). On the genesis of glaucoma. An improved method based on slit-lamp microscopy of the angle of the anterior chamber. *Am. J. Ophthalmol.,* **19:** 209–215.

Becker, S. C. (1972). *Clinical Gonioscopy: A Text and Stereoscopic Atlas.* St Louis, C.V. Mosby.

Begg, I. S. (1969). Significance of goniohaemorrhage in heterochromic cyclitis. *Br. J. Ophthalmol.,* **53:** 1–8.

Bill, A., and Phillips, C. I. (1971). Uveoscleral drainage of aqueous humour in human eyes. *Exp. Eye Res.,* **12:** 275–281.

Braley, A. E., and Allen, L. (1951). Corneal contact prism and corneal contact lens for slit lamp biomicroscopic examination of peripheral and central fundus. *Trans. Am. Ophthalmol. Soc.,* **49:** 477–483.

Braley, A. E., and Allen, L. (1954). Gonioscopy in non-glaucomatous young eyes as a basis for evaluating changes in relation to glaucoma. *Acta. XVII Conc. Ophthalmol.,* 48–59.

Brown, S. V. L., Thomas, J. V., *et al.* (1985). Laser trabeculoplasty retreatment. *Am. J. Ophthalmol.,* **99:** 8–10.

Burian, H. M., and Allen, L. (1954). Speculum contact lens electrode for electroretinography. *Electroencephalography and Clinical Neurophysiology,* **6:** 509–511.

Burian, H. M., and Allen, L. (1955). Mechanical changes during accommodation observed by gonioscopy. *Arch. Ophthalmol.,* **54:** 66–72.

Burian, H. M., and Allen, L. (1961). Histologic study of the chamber angle of patients with Marfan's syndrome. A discussion of the cases of Theobald, Rech and Lehman, and Sadide Buen and Velazquez. *Arch. Ophthalmol.,* **65:** 323–333.

Burian, H. M., Braley, A. E., *et al.* (1954). External and gonioscopic visibility of ring of Schwalbe and trabecular zone; interpretation of posterior corneal embryotoxon and so-called congenital hyaline membranes on posterior corneal surface. *Trans. Am. Ophthalmol. Soc.,* **52:** 389–428.

Burian, H. M., Rice, M. H., *et al.* (1957). External visibility of the region of Schlemm's canal. *Arch. Ophthalmol.,* **57:** 651–658.

Campbell, D. G. (1979). Pigmentary dispersion and glaucoma: a new theory. *Arch. Ophthalmol.,* **97:** 1667–1672.

Campbell, D. G. (1984). Iris retraction associated with rhegmatogenous retinal detachment syndrome and hypotony. *Arch. Ophthalmol.,* **102:** 1457–1463.

Campbell, D. G., Simmons, R. J., *et al.* (1976). Ghost cells as a cause of glaucoma. *Am. J. Ophthalmol.,* **81:** 441–450.

Chandler, P. A., and Grant, W. M. (1965). *Lectures on Glaucoma.* Philadelphia, Lea & Febiger.

Conte, J. E. (1986). Infection with human immunodeficiency virus in the hospital. *Ann. Int. Med.,* **105:** 730–736.

Dellaporta, A. (1975). Historical notes on gonioscopy. *Surv. Ophthalmol.,* **20:** 137–149.

Douvas, N., and Allen, L. (1950). Anterior segment photography with Nordenson retinal camera. *Am. J. Ophthalmol.,* **33:** 291–292.

Epstein, D. L. (1986). *Chandler and Grant's Glaucoma.* Philadelphia, Lea & Febiger.

Epstein, D. L., Jedziniak, J. A., *et al.* (1978). Identification of heavy-molecular-weight soluble protein in aqueous humor in human phacolytic glaucoma. *Invest. Ophthalmol. Vis. Sci.,* **17:** 398–402.

Flocks, M. (1956). The anatomy of the trabecular meshwork as seen in tangential section. *Arch. Ophthalmol.,* **56:** 708–718.

Forbes, M. (1966). Gonioscopy with indentation: a method for distinguishing between appositional closure and synechial closure. *Arch. Ophthalmol.,* **76:** 488.

Gabelt, B. T., and Kaufman, P. L. (1989). $PGF_{2\alpha}$ increases uveoscleral outflow in monkeys. *Exp. Eye Res.,* **49:** 389–402.

Gass, J. D. M. (1967). Retinal detachment and narrow-angle glaucoma secondary to inflammatory pseudotumor of the uveal tract. *Am. J. Ophthalmol.,* **64:** 612–621.

Goldmann, H. (1938). Zur Technik der Spaltlampenmikroskopie. *Ophthalmologica,* **96:** 90–97.

Gorin, G., and Posner, A. (1967). *Slit Lamp Gonioscopy.* Baltimore, Williams and Wilkins.

Gradle, H. S., and Sugar, H. S. (1940). Concerning the anterior chamber angle. III. A clinical method of goniometry. *Am. J. Ophthalmol.*, **23:** 1135–1139.

Grant, W. M., and Walton, D. S. (1974). Progressive changes in the angle in congenital aniridia with development of glaucoma. *Am. J. Ophthalmol.*, **78:** 842–847.

Grierson, I., and Chisholm, I. A. (1978). Clearance of debris from the iris through the drainage of the rabbit's eye. *Br. J. Ophthalmol.*, **62:** 694–704.

Henkind, P. (1964). Angle vessels in normal eyes: a gonioscopic evaluation and anatomic correlation. *Br. J. Ophthalmol.*, **48:** 551–557.

Hoffmann, F., and Dumitrescu, L. (1971). Schlemm's canal under the scanning electron microscope. *Ophthalmic Res.*, **2:** 37–45.

Hoskins, H. D., and Kass, M. (1989). *Becker–Shaffer's Diagnosis and Therapy of the Glaucomas.* St Louis, C.V. Mosby.

Jorizzo, P. A., Samples, J. R., *et al.* (1988). The effect of repeat argon laser trabeculoplasty. *Am. J. Ophthalmol.*, **106:** 682–685.

Judisch, G. F., Phelps, C. D., *et al.* (1979). Rieger's syndrome – a case report with a 15-year follow-up. *Arch. Ophthalmol.*, **97:** 2120–2122.

Kaufman, J. H., and Tolpin, D. W. (1974). Glaucoma after traumatic angle recession – a ten-year prospective study. *Am. J. Ophthalmol.*, **78:** 648–654.

Kimura, R. (1974). *Color Atlas of Gonioscopy.* Tokyo, Igaku Shorin Ltd.

Kimura, S. J., Hogan, M. J., *et al.* (1955). Fuchs' syndrome of heterochromic cyclitis. *Arch. Ophthalmol.*, **54:** 179–186.

Koeppe, L. (1919). Die Mikroskopie des lebenden Kammerwinkels im fokalen Lichte der Gullstrandschen Nernstspaltlampe. *Albrecht von Graefes Arch. Ophthalmol.*, **101:** 48–66.

Krachmer, J. H. (1985). Posterior polymorphous corneal dystrophy: a disease characterized by epithelial-like endothelial cells which influence management and prognosis. *Trans. Am. Ophthalmol. Soc.*, **83:** 413–475.

Lee, O. S., and Allen, L. (1949). Keratoplasty: preliminary report on development of instruments. *Am. J. Ophthalmol.*, **32:** 71–78.

Maumenee, I. H., Kenyon, K. R., *et al.* (1977). Familial aniridia with preserved ocular function. *Am. J. Ophthalmol.*, **83:** 718–724.

McDonald, P. R., and Ashodian, M. J. (1959). Retained glass foreign bodies in the anterior chamber. *Am. J. Ophthalmol.*, **48:** 747–750.

Merritt, J. C. (1976). Transpupillary photocoagulation of the ciliary processes. *Ann. Ophthalmol.*, **8:** 325–328.

Mizuo (1914). Ein Verfahren zur Besichtigung der Kammerbucht. *Klin. Monatsbl. Augenheilkunde,* **52:** 561.

Moses, R. A., and Grodzki, W. J. (1977). The scleral spur and scleral roll. *Invest. Ophthalmol. Vis. Sci.*, **16:** 925–931.

O'Brien, C. S., Allen, J. H., *et al.* (1946). Evisceration with intrascleral implant (new technique). *Trans. Am. Ophthalmol. Soc.*, **44:** 296–303.

Palmberg, P. (1989). Gonioscopy. In: Ritch, R., Shields, M. B., *et al.*, eds., *The Glaucomas.* St Louis, C.V. Mosby.

Partamian, L. G. (1985). Treatment of a cyclodialysis cleft with argon laser photocoagulation in a patient with a shallow anterior chamber. *Am. J. Ophthalmol.*, **99:** 5–7.

Pavlin, C. J., Ritch, R., *et al.* (1992). Ultrasound biomicroscopy in plateau iris syndrome. *Am. J. Ophthalmol.*, **113:** 390–395.

Pederson, J. E. (1986). Ocular hypotony. *Trans. Ophthalmol. Soc. UK,* **105:** 220–226.

Posner, A., and Schlossman, A. (1948). Syndrome of unilateral recurrent attacks of glaucoma with cyclitic symptoms. *Arch. Ophthalmol.,* **39:** 517–535.

Raeder, J. (1923). Untersuchungen über die Lage und Dicke der Linse im menschlichen Auge bei physiologischen und pathologischen Zustanden, nach einer neuen Methode gemessen. *Arch. f. Ophthalmol.,* **112:** 29–63.

Ritch, R. (1985). A new lens for argon laser trabeculoplasty. *Ophthalmic Surg.,* **16:** 331–332.

Ritch, R., Shields, M. B., *et al.* (1989). *The Glaucomas.* St Louis, C.V. Mosby.

Robin, A. L., Pollack, I. P., *et al.* (1987). Effects of ALO 2145 on intraocular pressure following argon laser trabeculoplasty. *Arch. Ophthalmol.,* **105:** 646–650.

Rodrigues, M. C., Spaeth, G. L., *et al.* (1983). Iridoschisis associated with glaucoma and bullous keratopathy. *Am. J. Ophthalmol.,* **95:** 73–81.

Rodrigues, M. C., Spaeth, G. L., *et al.* (1982). Electron microscopy of argon therapy in phakic open angle glaucoma. *Ophthalmology,* **89:** 198–210.

Rouhiainen, H. J., Teräsvirta, M. E., *et al.* (1988). Peripheral anterior synechiae formation after trabeculoplasty. *Arch. Ophthalmol.,* **106:** 189–191.

Salzmann, M. (1914). Die Ophthalmoskopie der Kammerbucht. *Z. Augenheilkunde,* **31:** 1–19.

Salzmann, M. (1915). Nachtrag zu Ophthalmoskopie der Kammerbucht. *Z. Augenheilkunde,* **34:** 160–162.

Scheie, H. G. (1957). Width and pigmentation of the angle of the anterior chamber. *Arch. Ophthalmol.,* **58:** 510–512.

Shaffer, R. N. (1960). Gonioscopy, ophthalmoscopy, and perimetry. *Trans. Am. Acad. Ophthalmol. Otolaryngol.,* **64:** 112–125.

Shaffer, R. N. (1962). *Stereoscopic Manual of Gonioscopy.* St Louis, C.V. Mosby.

Shaw, B., and Lewis, R. (1986). Intraocular pressure elevation after pupillary dilation in open angle glaucoma. *Arch. Ophthalmol.,* **104:** 1185–1188.

Shields, M. B. (1992). *Textbook of Glaucoma.* Baltimore, Williams & Wilkins.

Shields, M. B., Buckley, E., *et al.* (1985a). Axenfeld–Rieger syndrome. A spectrum of developmental disorders. *Surv. Ophthalmol.,* **29:** 387–409.

Shields, M. B., Chandler, D. B., *et al.* (1985b). Intraocular cyclophotocoagulation. *Arch. Ophthalmol.,* **103:** 1731–1735.

Shields, M. B., and Klintworth, G. K. (1980). Anterior uveal melanomas and intraocular pressure. *Ophthalmology,* **87:** 503–517.

Skuta, G. L., Parrish, R. K., *et al.* (1987). Zonular dialysis during extracapsular cataract extraction in pseudoexfoliation syndrome. *Arch. Ophthalmol.,* **105:** 632–634.

Spaeth, G. L. (1971). The normal development of the human anterior chamber angle: a new system of grading. *Trans. Ophthalmol. Soc. UK,* **91:** 709–739.

Spaeth, G. L. (1977). Distinguishing between the normally narrow, the suspiciously shallow, and the particularly pathological, anterior chamber chamber angle. *Perspectives in Ophthalmology,* **1:** 205–214.

Spencer, W. H., Alvarado, J., *et al.* (1968). Scanning electron microscopy of human ocular tissues: trabecular meshwork. *Invest. Ophthalmol.,* **7:** 651–662.

Streeten, B. W., Li, Z.-Y., *et al.* (1992). Pseudoexfoliative fibrillopathy in visceral organs of a patient with pseudoexfoliation syndrome. *Arch. Ophthalmol.,* **110:** 1757–1762.

Tanchel, N. A., Aiken, D. G., *et al.* (1984). Correlation of segments of trabecular meshwork pigmentation and collector channels. *Invest. Ophthalmol. Vis. Sci.* (suppl.), **25**: 122.

Teekhasaenee, C., Ritch, R., *et al.* (1990). Ocular findings in oculodermal melanocytosis. *Arch. Ophthalmol.*, **108**: 1114–1120.

Thomas, J. V., Simmons, R. J., *et al.* (1982). Argon laser trabeculoplasty in the presurgical glaucoma patient. *Ophthalmology,* **89**: 187–197.

Thorburn, T. (1927). A gonioscopical study of anterior peripheral synechiae in primary glaucoma. S*venska Läkaresällskapets Handligar*, **53**: 252.

Tonjum, A. M. (1966). Gonioscopy in traumatic hyphema. *Acta Ophthalmologica,* **44**: 650–664.

Tornquist, R. (1956). Chamber depth in primary acute glaucoma. *Br. J. Ophthalmol.,* **40**: 421–429.

Tornquist, R. (1957). Corneal radius in primary acute glaucoma. *Br. J. Ophthalmol.,* **41**: 421–424.

Trantas, A. (1918). L'ophtalmoscopie de l'angle iridocornéen. *Arch. Ophtalmol. (Paris),* **36**: 257–276.

Trantas, A. (1907). Ophtalmoscopie de la région ciliaire et rétrociliaire. *Arch. Ophtalmol. (Paris),* **27**: 581–606.

Tripathi, R. C. (1968). Ultrastructure of Schlemm's canal in relation to aqueous outflow. *Exp. Eye Res.,* **7**: 335–341.

Troncoso, M. U. (1925). Gonioscopy with the electric ophthalmoscope. New York Academy of Medicine.

Troncoso, M. U. (1947). *Gonioscopy.* Philadelphia, F.A. Davis.

Van Herick, W., Shaffer, R. N., *et al.* (1969). Estimation of width of angle of anterior chamber. Incidence and significance of the narrow angle. *Am. J. Ophthalmol.,* **68**: 626–629.

Von Noorden, G. K., Allen, L., *et al.* (1959). A photographic method for the determination of the behavior of fixation. *Am. J. Ophthalmol.,* **48**: 511–514.

Watzke, R. C., and Allen, L. (1963). The Allen–Watzke corneal graft holder. *Trans. Am. Acad. Ophthalmol. Otolaryngol.,* **67**: 558–559.

Weiss, D. I., and Shaffer, R. N. (1972). Ciliary block (malignant) glaucoma. *Trans. Am. Acad. Ophthalmol. Otolaryngol.,* **76**: 450–461.

Wise, J. B., and Witter, S. L. (1979). Argon laser therapy for open angle glaucoma. *Arch. Ophthalmol.,* **97**: 319–322.

Wolter, J. R., Sandall, G. S., *et al.* (1967). Mesodermal dysgenesis of anterior eye with a partially separated posterior embryotoxon. *J. Pediatr. Ophthalmol. Strabismus,* **4**: 41–46.

Wong, D., and Fishman, M. (1990). Lee Allen – the man, the legend. *J. Ophth. Photogr.,* **12**: 51–67.

Worst, J. G. F. (1966). *The Pathogenesis of Congenital Glaucoma.* Assen, Netherlands, Charles C. Thomas.

Yanoff, M. (1970). Glaucoma mechanisms in ocular malignant melanomas. *Am. J. Ophthalmol.,* **70**: 898–904.

Index

Numbers in **bold** refer to illustration page numbers

microspherophakia, 76
pigment dispersion syndrome, 87
unilateral high, 40

N
neovascularization, 48, **78-9**
  Fuchs' heterochromic iridocyclitis, **97-8**

O
ocular ischemia, 78
oculodermal melanocytosis, 91, **92**
outflow, aqueous, 12-4

P
panretinal photocoagulation, 85
periumbilical skin, redundant, 64
phacolytic glaucoma, **99-100**
pigment in angle, 33, **42-4**, 51, **87-93**
pigment dispersion syndrome, 39, **87-9**, 113
pilocarpine, 34, 49, 71
plateau iris, 39, **71, 72**, 115
polycoria
  essential iris atrophy, **80**
  Rieger's anomaly, **63**
Posner lens, **23**, 29
  indentation gonioscopy, 35-37
posterior embryotoxon, 46, **60-3**
posterior polymorphous dystrophy (PPMD), **80-1**
posterior pressure, 84
precipitates on trabecular meshwork, **95**, 97-8
primary infantile glaucoma, 20, **57-9**
primary open angle glaucoma, 87
pseudoexfoliation, 39, **90-1**, 113-4
pseudophakia, angle width, 48
pupillary block
  dislocated lens, **74-5**
  distinction from malignant glaucoma, 72-3
  primary angle closure, **36-8, 67-73**
  secondary, 73, **74-86**

R
recessed angle, 40, 47, 49, **103**
reflection, total internal, **17**
retinal detachment, 78, 111
retinal vein occlusion, 78
retinopathy of prematurity, 78
Rieger's anomaly, 61, **62, 63**
Rieger's syndrome, 61, **63-4**
Ritch lens, 20, **21**, 28, 113
rubeosis iridis, 48, **78-9, 97-8**

S
Salzmann, Maximilian, 15, **16**
Sampaolesi's line, 33, **43-4**, 46, 88
Scheie grading system, **51**
Scheie's stripe, **89**
Schlemm's canal, 9, 11, **12**, 13, **14**, 45
  blood in, 15, 20, 28, **45, 84, 94, 101, 107**
Schwalbe's line, 9, **11-2, 14**, 42-3, **45-6**

Axenfeld-Rieger's syndrome, **61-4**
Axenfeld's anomaly, **61-2**
corneal wedge, **30-4**
pigmentation, **33, 43-4**, 46, 48
posterior embryotoxon, 46, **60-3**
prominent, 46, **60-3, 84, 107**
scleral spur, **9, 11-2, 41**, 49
scleral sulcus, **11**
sclerostomy, patent internal, 107, **108**
setons, 107, **108**
Shaffer grading technique, 16, **52**
sickle cell disease, 78
siderosis, **101**
slit-lamp gonioscopy
  history, 16
  lenses, **21-4**
  principles, 20-5
  technique, 27-38
Sondermann's canals, 13
Spaeth grading system, 52, **53**
Sturge-Weber syndrome, 107
suprachoroidal hemorrhage, 73
surgery, angle changes, **107-11**
Sussman lens, 23, **24**, 29
  indentation gonioscopy, 35-37
Swan-Jacobs lens, **19, 20**, 57, **58**
synechiae, central posterior, 73, **74**
synechiae, peripheral anterior, **33, 35, 37**, 41, 47, **70**, 76, **77-83**
  after argon laser trabeculoplasty, 81, **83**
  after surgery, **81-3**
  after trauma, 81, **82**
  breaking, 77
  differentiated from iris processes, 47
  inflammatory, **77-8**, 83
  iridocorneal-endothelial syndromes, 79, **80**
  neovascularization, **78-9**
  posterior polymorphous dystrophy (PPMD), 80, **81**

T
tear-air interface, 17
Thorburn, 16
total internal reflection, **17**
trabecular meshwork, **9, 11-4, 42-4**
  age effects, 42
  endothelial cells, **13-4**
  inflammatory precipitates, **95**, 97-8
  lens particles on, **99**
  macrophage obstruction, **100**
  pigmentation, **42-4**, 87-93
  pillars, **13**
  precipitation syndrome, **95**, 97-8
  protein obstruction, 100
trabecular outflow, 12
trabecular pillars, 59, **100**
trabeculectomy, **73**, 107, **108**
trabeculoplasty, 81, **83**, 113, **114**, 115
transpupillary photocoagulation, **116**

Trantas, Alexios, **15**
trauma
  angle recession, 40, 47, 49, **103**
  blood in anterior chamber, **94-5**
  cyclodialysis, 35, 40, 49, **104**, 105
  foreign bodies in anterior chamber, **100-1**
  iridodialysis, **102**
Trokel lens, **22**, 28
Troncoso, Manuel Uribe, 16
tumors, **105-6**, **112**
U
umbilicus in Rieger's syndrome, **64**
Unger fork, **22**
uveal meshwork, 12
uveitis, chronic granulomatous, **77-8**

uveoscleral outflow, 11

V
van Herick estimation system, 25, 54, **55**
vitreous body
  in cataract wound, **110**
  pupillary block from, **76**
vitreous hemorrhage, ghost-cell glaucoma, 95

Weill-Marchesani syndrome, 76
Wilms' tumor, 64